The Secret Therapy of Trees

MARCO MENCAGLI AND MARCO NIERI

TRANSLATED BY JAMIE RICHARDS

RODALE

NEW YORK

The Secret Therapy of Trees

HARNESS THE HEALING ENERGY OF FOREST BATHING
AND NATURAL LANDSCAPES

Translation copyright © 2019 by Penguin Random House LLC

All rights reserved.

Published in the United States by Rodale Books, an imprint of Random House, a division of Penguin Random House LLC, New York.
rodalebooks.com

RODALE and the Plant colophon are registered trademarks of Penguin Random House LLC.

Originally published in Italy as *La Terapia Segreta Degli Alberi* by Sperling & Kupfer Editori S.p.A. in 2017, copyright © 2017 by Sperling & Kupfer Editori S.p.A., copyright © 2018 by Mondadori Libri S.p.A. for the imprint Sperling & Kupfer.

Library of Congress Cataloging-in-Publication Data
Names: Mencagli, Marco, author.
Title: The secret therapy of trees / Marco Mencagli and Marco Nieri.
Other titles: Terapia segreta degli alberi. English
Description: New York: Rodale Books, [2018] | "Originally published in Italy by Sperling & Kupfer Editori S.p.A in 2016."
Identifiers: LCCN 2018060078 | ISBN 9781984824141 (hardcover) | ISBN 9781984824158 (ebook)
Subjects: LCSH: Trees—Therapeutic use. | Plants—Therapeutic use. | Human beings—Effect of environment on. | Nature, Healing power of.
Classification: LCC QK99.A1 M4613 2018 | DDC 582.16—dc23
LC record available at https://lccn.loc.gov/2018060078

ISBN 978-1-9848-2414-1
Ebook ISBN 978-1-9848-2415-8

Printed in the United States of America

Book design by Elina Nudelman
Tree art by NikhomTreeVector/Shutterstock
Cover design by Sarah Horgan
Cover illustration by Nikhom TreeVector/Shutterstock

Illustrations on pages 137 and 143 appear courtesy of the author.
Illustration that appears on page 145 is copyright © 2019 by Kirlionics Technologies International.

10 9 8 7 6 5 4 3 2 1

First U.S. Edition

To T., with immense gratitude and admiration

To A., the splendid sunflower
that I met on my path, with love

CONTENTS

The Secret Therapy of Trees

In light of the research on nature's restorative benefits on our physical and emotional health, we can all agree that being in touch with nature is closely connected to our well-being. We're instinctively drawn toward green spaces, even if we aren't aware of the reasons why. Yet now more than ever, it's not enough to be content with knowing that nature is good for us. It's a notion as obvious as it is too readily underestimated.

In many countries with advanced economies, over the last century their "arboreal heritage" (not only woodland) has been rising. In the United States, along with certain European countries, reserved forestland has doubled from the nation's birth to today.

Given this decidedly positive fact, which goes against the general trend shown in world data, we all need to pay more attention to the importance of green space—and nature in general—to take advantage of all that it has to offer for the betterment of our health and well-being. We must also try to understand that there are places and circumstances in which nature really can do *so much* for our well-being.

But let's take a step back. In the United States, over 80 percent of the population lives in urban and suburban areas (those with a population density equal to or above five hundred inhabitants per square mile), and less than 20 percent lives in rural areas. In industrialized European countries, these percentages are similar, and in some cases, the discrepancy is even greater.

While it's true that in the last century the size of the forests and wooded areas in the United States has grown to cover over one third of the country's entire surface, it's also true that the U.S. population has more than tripled in the same period. In fact, for some countries, population growth has actually corresponded to a major decrease in natural green space.

We should not, then, be surprised by the emergence of a widespread "need for nature" that has no precedent in history. Numerous scientific and sociological studies explain this well, demonstrating how important it is for contemporary humankind to maintain or resume contact with the natural environment that has been the evolutionary cradle of the species. And yet we adopt behaviors that seem to take us in the opposite direction every day.

Our coexistence with nature has dwindled with the rise of lifestyles that are filled with pressing commitments and highly dependent on technology, leading to unhealthy levels of stress and the resulting health problems. This is the very reason why we need to be in contact with nature.

Conscious of this shift, architects, designers, and professionals in travel and leisure increasingly offer spaces and experiences that make it possible to live in direct contact with green space.

However, the recent rediscovery of nature is often superficial. We've found a way to commodify nature, consuming it in the limited amount of free time we can find in our workday or on the weekend, or, in the best case, on vacation.

We know that no matter how brief, these interactions are a step in the right direction. Nevertheless, we need to learn how to make the most of the natural spaces around us. By knowing how to tap into the world around us, we can fix the damage done by our urban lifestyles.

Within these pages, you'll discover why nature's absence from our daily lives is causing serious social damage and how exposure to nature can help us to alleviate recurring pains and anxieties. You'll also learn how to tap into the great therapeutic potential of green space, potential that has remained largely unexplored and accessible only to a select few, as if for some reason the potential were intentionally kept a secret.

As it happens, there is no big secret to "reveal," only an understanding of how we can foster our daily well-being by incorporating nature into our lives—from the forest to the houseplant on your desk.

This is the most comprehensive look at the noticeable improvements that trees, plants, and greenery in general can enact on our bodies and minds.

Forest therapy or *forest medicine* is already an emerging therapeutic approach used by psychologists, biologists, physicians, and health-care workers, who draw on interdisciplinary research and experience to identify the great beneficial power of nature and green space. The most innovative research includes studies of the effects of aromatic substances (monoterpenes) issued by trees on the immune system, and of the presence of negative ions, beneficial to health, in the atmosphere of certain settings. The frontiers of knowledge and experimentation have even opened up to the subtle electromagnetic relationships between the biosphere and living beings, revealing how trees can interact with humans on the bioenergetic level and increase individual well-being.

Using the concepts and methods described in this book, you can turn any act associated with nature into an effective means of therapy, from a simple walk to more targeted practices of psychophysical rehabilitation and care, whether hortitherapy, nature therapy, ecotherapy, or coaching or brainstorming sessions conducted in green space. Doing so will result in lower levels of stress (which can have so many physical repercussions), and even lower risks of heart disease and cancer.

As experts who have been enthusiastically exploring these areas for years, we want to share our knowledge and offer concrete aid in consciously recognizing and utilizing the support that nature provides for our health.

"Knowledge" and "consciousness" are, in fact, key words, both for reminding us who we are and where we come from, and for rediscovering the value of the natural environment we live in. The natural world can give us much more than mere entertainment or an escape from chemical, sound, or visual pollutants.

Going forest bathing, finding trees that interact with us on the energetic level, or even just bringing plants into the home or workplace is in itself an important step toward reconnecting with our roots and a profound act of self-care.

We hope you enjoy the journey.

Happy reading!

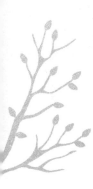

1. NATURE'S IMPRINT: IS IT TRULY FOREVER?

It's not so hard to admit: our contact with nature has become increasingly rare. Not exactly breaking news. Life moves on regardless . . . maybe not exactly how we would like, but it does.

Unfortunately, this mind-set minimizes the problem at hand. We like nature, we know it's important for our well-being, but we don't give it a central role in our lives. This is a generalization, of course. Even in today's hypertechnological world, some of us think and act differently. In fact, there are young people who are returning to rural life, an indication of the trend toward ecological and environmental sensitivity. Still, they are the minority.

In 2009, the world's population surpassed 6.8 million: that was the year in which, for the first time, city dwellers outnumbered rural residents, an occurrence that the Worldwatch

Institute had predicted for 2008. Demographers have shown that this trend will continue to rise. The latest forecasts hypothesize that by the year 2030 approximately 75 percent of the world's population will live in urban areas.

While Europe and North America have already reached this percentage, the rest of the world is racing to urbanize. There are at least twenty (or twice that, if greater metropolitan areas are considered) world megalopoli, cities with over ten million inhabitants, at least two of which are in Africa.

It's time to start examining how our relationship to nature has been affected in light of this societal shift, instead of passively accepting our circumstances. At the root of our substantial indifference to this situation, as we must acknowledge, is a certain desire not to know. It's similar to the attitude many have toward events of vast social significance: when faced with issues we find too difficult, we prefer to hand the problem to someone else. But leaving the decision up to others could have disastrous consequences.

Some people, for example, provocatively assert that all this attention on environmental issues and humanity's relationship to nature is just a fad. Others believe we should establish a new bond with the natural world: something more technical, more geared toward extracting benefits based on cause and effect, where nature becomes a tool (not to say a consumer product) for self-improvement. We respectfully disagree: something inside us, a little voice, tells us that can't be right. But what is the source of that voice? Perhaps it's the part of us that conserves the historic (or rather, genetic) memory of who we are and where we come from.

So that's where we should start.

For a very long time, natural environments have been our habitat, or, to be more precise, our *home.* At first, we were humble occupants, then we resolved to become ambitious dominators. Here are some facts to consider—the genus *Homo* has existed on Earth for 2.3 to 2.4 million years, according to the latest anthropological studies. And the more "human" variant of the genus *Homo,* the one that most resembles us, has been given an age of approximately 1 million years, more or less coinciding with the time that they learned to use fire.

The species *Homo sapiens* formed just under two hundred thousand years ago on the continent of Africa, the same place where their ancestors-predecessors originated. When *Homo sapiens* appeared, *Homo erectus* also existed in Asia, and *Homo neanderthalensis* in Europe. *Homo erectus* went extinct soon thereafter, while we know that at least forty to fifty thousand years ago Sapiens encountered—and for a short time lived alongside—Neanderthals, before the latter went extinct in turn.

After their appearance on the planet, Sapiens briefly remained in their place of origin, Africa, but within a hundred thousand years they had colonized the Middle East and from there moved onto other lands: Southeast Asia, Europe, Oceania, and America.

For a very long time, the first representatives of the *Homo* genus were gatherers and then hunters, living off what nature was able to offer more or less spontaneously. The shift to agricultural society, which happened gradually, was unique to *Homo sapiens.* In fact, the first "professional" farmers emerged just eleven thousand years ago. Once human beings began devoting themselves to agriculture, their dwellings shifted from the forests. After all, hunter-gatherer villages contained only a few dozen people, while those of a farming society could easily exceed a hundred. These new communities required more space.

The first true cities, with hundreds of inhabitants, arose just over eight thousand years ago. (It is estimated that the world's population at the time was no more than seven to eight million—a very modest number compared with, for example, the buffalo population then living on the North American plains.) Over the course of the next eight thousand years, the rise in urban population essentially never saw a downturn.

These few figures are enough to establish with some certainty that—as the beginning of the agricultural age ushered in the definitive retreat from the forests and savannas—man as a species has spent 99.5 percent of his evolutionary time in completely natural environments. Even today, a portion of the world's population spends their entire existence there. Perhaps a bit loosely, we "civilized" humans tend to define these environments as "green space," sometimes imprecisely alongside the expression "untouched by man." Let us remember, however, that our species lived in these places—and *only* in these places—up until, in relation to the entire history of our species, what amounts to a few moments ago.

It is therefore possible that our own evolutionary history is what drives us to love green spaces, even in the context of contemporary living. There are several fascinating examples that illustrate this theory, on both the emotional and behavioral level.

Our Unbreakable Bond with Nature

The scientific community is still unable to definitively determine how many colors the human eye can perceive. Various biomedical reports show numbers ranging from a minimum of 100,000 to a theoretical maximum of 10 million shades. Yet there is a consensus (and study results) that green is the color for which humans can distinguish the greatest number of shades. The difference is significant: for green it's about 100 hues, while for other colors, including composite colors, it's only a few dozen. This phenomenon has evolutionary origins.

Green is the most common color in nature, as it is the typical pigment color of chlorophyll, which is present in all primitive and evolved plant species that use the process of photosynthesis. The ancestors of *Homo sapiens*, certainly not one of the strongest mammals on the planet physically, quickly learned to discern the various shades of green in vegetation, deciphering the elements of the surrounding environment in order to increase their chances of survival. This behavioral adaptation translated into a morphological and physiological adaptation of our "warning system": an imprint of nature that has remained with us up to the present.

Even more surprising are the differences between reaction times at the sudden appearance of an animal or a moving object, such as a car. Recent studies conducted at the University of California, Santa Barbara, have shown that those who live in urban environments, no doubt more used to navigating the dangers of traffic and moving vehicles, demonstrate much shorter reaction times at the sight of an animal than an automobile suddenly appearing in their field of vision.

Equally noted are the several experiments conducted on small children who had never been exposed to potentially dangerous animals such as spiders or snakes. Even if the children couldn't understand the threat from a cognitive perspective, they showed a physiological response to the stress of merely viewing images of such animals.

Analogous experiments have been conducted using sophisticated camouflage techniques to show adults images of potentially dangerous animals (like spiders) in rapid succession interspersed with neutral objects, such as flowers and mushrooms, so that the subject did not consciously perceive the stimuli. Electroencephalograms regularly registered stress responses at the sight of the threatening stimuli, a sign that "ancient fears" are well rooted in the subconscious and show greater resistance to repression than other modern threats, like guns or knives.

Similar studies focusing on our sense of hearing confirm that human beings register and decipher nature sounds differently than those connected with modern life. For example, one might assume that an alarm created by a rapid series of high-pitched sounds (typical for danger signals) would trigger an alert response very quickly. However, a study published in 2011 in the *Journal of the Acoustical Society of America* demonstrated that people react fastest to the sounds of animal predators, like the lion, tiger, or jaguar, rather than to common artificial alarms. Of course, that doesn't mean that using a lion roar for a home security alarm would be more effective in deterring unwanted visitors, though it would be an interesting experiment.

On the other hand, natural noises such as water flowing down a stream or birds chirping can mask our auditory perception of street traffic and other noises typical of urban environments. Indeed, the introduction of nature sounds seems to diminish the disturbance of artificial noises, especially in indoor work environments.

Humans, evidently, always prefer to hear sounds that come from nature.

Biophilia

Human beings' innate tendency to prefer natural places and sounds, and to be curious about, attracted to, or at least attentive to other living creatures can be explained with the concept of biophilia.

Coined at the beginning of the twentieth century with a meaning slightly different from current usage, the term "biophilia" was revived in the mid-1980s by Harvard University biologist/entomologist Edward O. Wilson (the father of sociobiology) to describe our "innate tendency to focus on life and life-like processes." "Biophilia" is defined as "the innately emotional affiliation of human beings to other living organisms."

The concept of biophilia represents the idea that human beings, having evolved in places on the planet rich in plant and animal species, possess a deep biological attraction to what we identify today with the generic term "nature." This affinity with nature and everything that comprises it is therefore a product of natural selection. After Wilson, many other scholars have hypothesized (and later demonstrated) that the human predisposition to appreciate nature is genetic in origin. When we speak of nature's "imprint" on certain human behaviors and instinctive reactions, we're referring precisely to the genetic matrix of these influences. An obvious example of this genetic influence is the fact that individuals coming from different cultures and countries far removed from each other geographically show a preference for similar types of living space. These are real "environmental archetypes" humans have carried inside them for a very long time.

To get an idea of what these model habitats might be, we need to start once again with Edward Wilson, in his book *The Future of Life*: "Studies conducted in . . . environmental psychology during the past thirty years point consistently to the following conclusion: people prefer to be in natural environments, and especially in savanna or parklike habitats. They like a long depth of view across a relatively smooth, grassy ground surface dotted with trees and copses. They want to be near a body of water, whether ocean, lake, river, or stream. They try to place their habitations on a prominence, from which they can safely scan the savanna and watery environment. With nearly absolute consistency these landscapes are preferred over urban settings that are either bare or clothed in scant vegetation."

The author specifies that not all natural environments hold the same appeal: "To a relative degree people dislike woodland views that possess restricted depth of vision, a disordered complexity of vegetation, and rough ground structures—in short, forests with small, closely spaced trees and dense undergrowth. They want a topography and openings that improve their line of sight." From there it's easy to conclude that similar preferences would have been shown by the progenitors of *Homo sapiens*.

Various studies arrive at these same observations; there are two worth mentioning in particular. In a work published in 1993, Professor Roger Ulrich of Texas A&M University reports that among the various models of natural landscapes that his research subjects were shown, those categorized as savanna were more strongly associated with a calm and peaceful state of mind. Another American study, by John D. Balling and John H. Falk, found that this preference is even more marked in small children, who are less conditioned by familiarity with certain models.

This research aimed to examine the preferences of different age groups for five different types of environmental models (savanna, deciduous forest, temperate coniferous forest, equatorial rainforest, and desert). The results show a significant preference for the savanna environment by children from eight to eleven; older children, on the other hand, chose equally the savanna and the deciduous forest (a habitat with which they'd had more direct experience). These two environments turned out to be far preferred to the other three: it seems the evolutionary imprint is strongest in childhood, while as we get older cultural factors intervene and direct our choice toward more familiar environments.

A Relationship Adrift?

Given humanity's innate preference for natural environments, the phenomenon of urbanization is having increasingly noticeable results, certainly not limited to issues of mental and physical well-being.

We now know that from a biological perspective, we are not so different from our ancestors, and nature's imprint on our most instinctual behaviors is still very strong. It is a "genetic heritage" developed over hundreds of thousands of years, and appears even in contemporary lifestyles that no longer have anything in common with a life spent in the forest or savanna. But no one is certain whether in the future this imprint will be replaced by another or will disappear, in whole or in part.

Certain signs, however, should give us pause. One is our tendency toward environmental neglect. Living in places with minimal (or even nonexistent) greenery prevents us from coming into contact with more natural ways of living, to the point where we consider them impossible to pursue or perceive them distortedly.

When environmental neglect is the most common sight around us, it's easy to get used to the mind-set that there is no viable alternative, and thus the only solution is to adapt. But reducing our sensitivity to a situation that implicitly creates chronic stress is not the solution. We'll return to this subject further on. What we want to point out here is that we pay a price for these mechanisms of adaptation—for example, the loss of empathy for natural environments and the resulting emergence of a number of unhealthy behaviors that in turn become unhealthy habits.

Another disturbing sign is the "city kid's" aversion to natural settings. It might be amusing to see a kid frightened at the sight of a farm animal like a chicken or duck that has turned out to be a little too "lively." But if we really think about it, it's not a laughing matter: it is, sadly, a specific symptom of our changed lifestyles, as is a lack of interest in taking a walk through the forests or wooded areas or just climbing a tree. These activities are often replaced by excessive attention to phones, TVs, and computers. This behavior shows that different lifestyles can affect our natural imprint, or more precisely, our innate preference for habitats that "contain" nature.

Similar observations have led to the formulation of a constructivist theory stating that enjoyment of natural environments is not merely innate, but reinforced by attitudes acquired in early childhood, where the most formative and fun play takes place in the outdoors. During these activities, natural elements (trees, flowers, fields, animals, etc.) actively participate in constructing an individual's cognitive background, which will leave a long-term impression on his cultural memory.

In this way, an affective and emotional bond with nature is established. We don't view nature as "other," but rather as part of ourselves. This is an essential aspect in children's character development, with implications that they will carry with them for the rest of their lives.

In general, children appreciate green space immensely. Nature acts as a gym for a less structured (and thus more free) type of play that improves motor skills, fosters creative development, and enables learning to explore. Various studies have shown that spending time in parks and other "friendly" natural settings stimulates children's cognitive abilities over the long term at both the preschool and grade-school age.

The study also showed a continuation of heightened environmental sensibility, even as the subjects reached adulthood. Furthermore, if children are accustomed to fully appreciating the value of natural environments, they will retain this positive way of relating to nature as adults, which benefits them mentally as well as physically.

So what are we waiting for? Get yourself (and your kids, if you have them) to the park and keep reading!

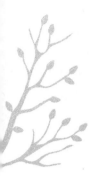

2. IS NATURE'S APPEAL FADING?

Let's try a little meditation exercise. This is a simple exercise many will already know, which requires no physical or mental preparation. The only tool we need is our attention.

First, find a park or any other natural or seminatural environment that you like and that is easily accessible. It would be a good idea to repeat this exercise whenever possible, until it becomes a positive habit when you visit "your" green space. For now, going to the nearest park will suffice.

This practice requires no more than a few minutes. Treat it as a brief, welcome pause in the activities of your daily life, that doesn't compromise your plans for the day.

Once you've found a place, you should find a vantage point where you can observe the whole setting and various details of the surrounding environment. Rather than acting merely as a spectator, imagine being the owner of that green space and the only one who truly and deeply understands its value.

For the first minute, look closely at your surroundings. Perhaps there are elements you don't like or that don't meet your taste, but turn your attention to focus on the things that attract you the most.

Now comes the work. Admiring or even just appreciating the place you're in isn't enough: you want to make a memory that's truly your own, a perspective that is completely personal and thus unique. So how do you do that? Take a few mental pictures, intended for yourself, to keep the memory of this encounter alive. To make sure that you don't forget them, imagine that your "mental camera" is out of memory and there is only room for three pictures, with no way to free up space to store more. You'll need to choose carefully: the three most beautiful scenes, the ones that best represent the space in front of you.

Free your mind of all else.

For the next five minutes, your sole task is to choose three of the many possible images with which you will create your own personal memory of the green space you're in. These will be the three images you'll carry along inside you and can happily recall any time you want.

As happens whenever we take an important photograph, we activate our consciousness and take in the breadth of our view, the depth of the field, the details, the light and shadow, the contrasts and tones . . . And what draws our attention might be the shape of a tree or bush, the softness of a patch of grass, the color contrasts between flowers or foliage of different plant species, the background created by the blue of the sky or the shape of the clouds, the presence of children playing or the solitude of the place. The details are very important; they make up a unique picture that we realize may only last a few moments.

First shot.

Change of frame. Once again, the choice falls on one or more details that you hadn't noticed before.

Second shot.

Another important view to imprint onto your mind.

Third shot.

Close your eyes for a moment and bring your three photographs back to the surface of your mind. Acknowledge the work you just did and feel satisfied.

The exercise finishes here. For three long moments, whether consciously or not, you meditated on the beauty of a natural place and tried to preserve its memory, cultivating your innate sense of belonging to it.

You had a brief yet concrete natural experience.

Far from Negligible Effects

Some people might deem the above exercise useless and silly, and quickly set it aside. But this actually confirms a problematic aspect of our relationship with nature: the superficiality or distraction with which we approach our experience with green space. The systemic lack of information and knowledge of the experiences that these places make possible prevents us from consciously grasping their therapeutic and regenerative potential. A direct consequence is the growing disinterest in empathetically visiting natural environments, which in turn gives rise to the behaviors and habits with noticeable side effects on our physical and mental well-being.

To understand more clearly, consider these examples.

In many Anglophone countries, East Asia, and, more recently, Scandinavia, numerous studies have been conducted on the correlation between proximity to green space and health. These studies are useful because they go beyond the common conception that nature "is good for you" and supply data on precisely how much good it does. The results, often referring to large samples of the population, are very interesting.

In 2010, a group of researchers from several Danish universities led by Professor Ulrika K. Stigsdotter published a study in the *Scandinavian Journal of Public Health* conducted on a sample of 11,238 citizens of Denmark. The goal of the study was to investigate not only the connection between green space and health but also the relationship between quality of life (related to health) and stress. The results of the investigation were truly remarkable: the interviewees who lived more than a kilometer away from green space (a park, forest, undeveloped lake or beach, etc.) had on average a 42 percent higher probability of feeling stressed compared with those who lived less than 300 meters away.

Furthermore, those in the first group who did not report symptomatic states of stress tended nonetheless to visit natural environments more often than subjects who would describe themselves as stressed. A vicious cycle revealed itself—people already under stress had less contact with nature, depriving themselves of a potential balancing factor and creating greater mental and physical disturbance. The interviewees who habitually visited green space indicated different reasons for seeking contact with nature: the desire for peace and tranquillity (and for the more stressed, peace of mind); opportunities for physical activity and staying in shape; and social occasions prevailed among those who were essentially in good health.

In any case, everyone agreed on the fact that regularly passing time in green space could promote good health; however, those who experienced stress tended to visit them less frequently on average. The results of this study follow those of analogous studies conducted in different parts of the world: from Australia to China, Japan to the United States, and Canada to Great Britain. They all confirmed the lower instance of death and serious illness (including heart disease and cancer) for those who live close to adequate green space.

These results have been confirmed over time thanks to the use of ever-more-sophisticated tools to gather and process data on the area and the population. A 2008 study, published in *The Open Public Health Journal* by a group of Japanese medical researchers led by Dr. Qing Li (one of the first to conduct research on the salutary practice of forest bathing), reported the results of a massive investigation conducted in every prefecture of Japan, showing a direct correlation, within a specific area, between a larger percentage of forest coverage and lower rates of cancer deaths. This correlation was significant particularly for uterine, breast, and lung cancers in the female population, and cancers of the prostate, liver, and colon in the male population.

The data on death rates from lung cancer in the female population of the Tokyo and Hiroshima Prefectures—which contain, respectively, 36 percent and 72 percent forest coverage within their territory—showed a 13 percent higher mortality rate in the prefecture with less surface area covered by forests. The difference in male deaths from prostate cancer is almost 20 percent. Both of these figures were statistically significant even after the necessary corrections were made for the number of smokers and population development indexes in each prefecture. Dr. Qing Li therefore asserted that a significant amount of forest area can contribute to a lower incidence of cancer.

There are many examples of large-scale studies, and we will look at others in later chapters. They have the merit of getting out of the closed laboratory environment to objectively measure the benefits of the presence and size of green spaces in specific areas, not merely the perceptions or impressions of those who live nearby or visit.

The overwhelming evidence suggests that the widespread and increasing departure from nature is not a potential but a concrete risk to our health.

Health in the Plural

"Health" does not refer only to the physical. In 1948, the World Health Organization came up with this still-pertinent definition of health: "state of complete physical, mental and social well-being and not merely the absence of disease or infirmity." Health must be assessed from multiple perspectives—physical, emotional, and even social health.

In support of one of those perspectives, many studies have shown the social (and even economic) advantages of having green spaces in urban settings.

In the minds of some, public parks are unsafe places, especially at night. This may be partially true if the architecture and landscape and type of vegetation in the park reduce visibility, if lighting is scarce or absent, or if there aren't many people visiting over the course of the day. Contrary to what we are led to believe, the presence of parks, gardens, and other green spaces in urban environments is statistically correlated with lower crime rates. Various studies conducted in urban areas of the United States (Chicago in 2001, and Portland, Oregon, in 2012) demonstrate this, placing crime data from police alongside percentage of green space in neighborhoods and larger areas. When comparing urban areas with little to no public or private green space with areas with high percentages of green space, especially trees, the total number of crimes (residential theft, robbery, and assault) was notably higher in the former. The correlation was very significant. In the Chicago study, for example, the lack of green space in a neighborhood corresponded to a more than 50 percent higher crime rate, at a peak of 56 percent in the category of "violent crime."

The data also confirms a well-known biological law, found among both animals and human beings: when individual space is reduced, antisocial behavior increases, displays of aggression worsen, and individualism triumphs over reciprocity. In a residential setting or habitat without sufficient outdoor space, especially for public use, there is often a severe breakdown in social relations, whereas seeing and visiting green spaces produces adaptive responses in people that facilitate relaxation and mitigate irritable states and mental fatigue.

The studies show two other fundamental elements of social health. The presence of tree-lined streets, lawns, and large green spaces at the neighborhood level encourages people to go outside and spend time in the open air, helping them overcome fears about the lack of safety in parks. With the level of surveillance increased by a higher number of visitors, the ill-intentioned are naturally discouraged. Furthermore, those who live near shared green space know their neighbors better and thus tend to socialize with them more, developing a sense of local belonging and social responsibility.

Other investigations with similar aims have also shown that nature acts as a "social equalizer," meaning that it is able to put groups of people from different socioeconomic backgrounds and geographic origins into contact with one another. In other words, when we find ourselves habitually frequenting green space, we will happily engage with others while sitting on a bench or taking a walk.

The "Screen Generation"

It's probably not unrealistic to state that today, for an increasing majority of the planet, the most often used everyday object is something with a screen. We don't mean to demonize the use of computers, smartphones, tablets, televisions, or other technological products, nor to underestimate their utility, but we must seriously reflect on the time we devote to these devices in relation to the time it takes away from our contact with nature.

Technology has allowed us to access much more information than we could even a few years ago, with huge advantages in all sectors of daily life. But the consumption of information is, as we know, a double-edged sword.

Statistics indicate that from 1980 to 2009 the consumption of nonwork-related information has risen over 450 percent: quite a "brain bomb," one could say. In Europe, the Eurostat agency reports that in domestic settings Internet access rose from 41 percent in 2004 to 83 percent in 2015.

A 2015 study on Internet use by adults in Great Britain found that:

- **96 percent of young adults between the ages of 16 and 24** (i.e., almost all) use the Internet when on the go (a figure that falls to 29 percent for those over 65), primarily using smartphones and tablets;

- **almost 61 percent of adults use social networks** (Twitter, Facebook, Instagram, etc.), and 79 percent report doing so every day or almost; this means that almost half of British adults use social networks on a near-daily basis;

- **76 percent of adults interviewed say they have purchased goods or services online during the last year** (in 2008 it was 53 percent), many to save time compared with a more traditional means of purchase. (Ideally the time saved went toward interaction with nature, but it's unlikely.)

The trends that emerge from this study are common to all technologically advanced countries. And there's more.

A recent study conducted in the United States showed that approximately 75 percent of employed adults between the ages of 18 and 44 state that they regularly check their work e-mail while on vacation. Great Britain is no better: a survey of 500 workers interviewed about their "tech" habits revealed that almost 60 percent look at their work e-mail while on vacation, while over 40 percent do it daily outside of working hours.

But an excessive use of electronic devices doesn't just affect the working world: a recent survey conducted by Durex on the habits of 2,000 adults on vacation found that 40 percent of interviewees were less likely to have sex if their partner was using a cell phone in bed; 41 percent admitted spending nights in bed with their partner with each of them on their smartphone rather than doing "something else." It's not a far leap from here to seeing how cell phone use can exclude nature from our lives.

Unsurprisingly, this dependence on technology has affected our behavioral preferences as well.

In 2010, the secretary of the Convention on Biological Diversity launched a survey of 10,000 children and adolescents between the ages of 5 and 18 in ten nations—1,000 from each of the selected nations: the United Kingdom, France, Germany, Spain, the United States, Japan, China, Mexico, Singapore, and Australia.

Asked to rank the things most important to them, around 40 percent of the children selected "watching TV or playing on the computer" as the most important, whereas "saving the environment" was chosen by only 4 percent.

In a study conducted at the beginning of 2012, two researchers from the University of Maryland School of Business showed that after brief mobile phone use, subjects were less inclined toward "prosocial behavior"—that is, actions aimed at helping society or other people—compared with the control group. The mobile phone users were also less engaged when responding to verbal tests, even knowing that correct answers would result in donations to charity.

According to the authors of the study, the use of mobile phones directly satisfies our sense of connectivity with others, saturating the natural sense of belonging needed by human beings. This explains the decreased desire to personally interact with neighbors or engage in empathetic or prosocial behavior. Along with this physical exclusion of others comes less empathy toward nature and our peers, self-centeredness, and loss of emotional intelligence. It also does not bode well for mental or physical well-being.

One of the primary sources of stress, both individually and collectively, is the excess of information to which we are all constantly subjected. If you're not stressed, you're likely in the minority. It's no coincidence that people are looking for that secret recipe to happiness. According to a recent study by former professor of medicine at Harvard Medical School Eva M. Selhub, more than three out of four books available for purchase on Amazon after the year 2000 had the word "happiness" in the title.

According to Dr. Selhub, we are searching for a way to overcome the now-common mental and physical distress that affects us when faced with particular recurring stimuli, such as numerous readily available sources of information.

In physiological terms, screen-projected images stimulate regions of the brain with densely packed dopamine receptors, dopamine being a neurotransmitter that has various functions in the body and which the brain produces as a reward for seeking out those things necessary for our survival such as food, water, physical activity, et cetera. The pleasure derived from satisfying a vital need is created by the release of dopamine in our brain. This is the result of a very powerful evolutionary mechanism. Humans have learned to expand the possibilities of experiencing this pleasure alongside their cultural evolution: even receiving a gift, for example, can activate this mechanism.

Thus, it seems our brain "interprets" an unread e-mail or an incoming cell phone message as a type of gift, a little surprise related to us personally and just waiting to be unwrapped.

Even the expectations that come from searching for information on the Internet function in the same way: our brains are constantly driven to release dopamine in response to stimuli coming from a screen.

Now let's try to think about how many messages we receive on our smartphone over the course of a day, and how many e-mails. Clearly, growing accustomed to an almost constant flow of dopamine in the brain leads to addiction.

At this point, we don't need to ask ourselves why it's so difficult to turn off the cell phone during the day even when we're on vacation, or why we can't do without checking our profiles on social networks even during work hours: work tasks burden us, producing stress that the brain interprets as a threat to our well-being. The posts in our social media feeds are little presents that release the dopamine reward we need at that moment. This also results, however, in growing difficulty in concentrating on our own activities, and a tendency to distraction and mental fatigue.

We feel more tired and more irritable, resulting in more stress. Reading work e-mail when we're on vacation is not just a type of workaholism: it's a symptom that we've more than likely developed an addiction. Turning our attention to cell phones and personal computers constantly so as not to feel "excluded from the party" leads us, in reality, to exclude much more important and concrete things, in addition to taking a signifi-cant quantity of time out of our day. This is not a recipe for happiness.

But there's good news: a better path exists. We've already caught a glimpse of it at the beginning of this chapter.

3. STRESS, IMMUNE DEFENSES, AND THE EXPERIENCE OF NATURE

We've already seen that regular, conscious, empathetic, and unrushed contact with nature can significantly help us to face the disturbances caused by stress, particularly many forms of chronic stress. The scientific literature demonstrating this effectiveness has been growing for decades and in numerous fields, from medicine and psychology to biology, biochemistry, and sociology, with increasing attention to the interdisciplinary.

But how does stress act in our body? What are the implications for our health?

We know that stress is a state of "activation" of certain bodily systems in response to stressors that are interpreted as threats (real or imagined) by the individual experiencing them. The entire body is involved, but most affected are the endocrine, circulatory, respiratory, digestive, and immune systems. The starting point, however, is in the nervous system, particularly in two specific regions of the brain.

When we think about stress, understood as a carrier of various maladies that can also seriously compromise our health, we only have the immediate vision of the pathology in mind. But the processes at the base of these physiological changes are actually evolutionary survival mechanisms.

All animals, even plants, are endowed with the ability to react and adapt to possibly dangerous stimuli in the environment. For example, some beetles, as well as certain vertebrates, have developed a behavior called thanatosis, or "playing dead." If they encounter something they interpret as dangerous, these insects stiffen up and appear to be dead. This is how they attempt to escape natural predators, who prefer to eat living or freshly killed prey and not decaying corpses. The common European grass snake (*Natrix natrix*) turns upside down with its mouth open in a rigid, unnatural pose and secretes a foul-smelling liquid that simulates decomposition.

The Hungarian-Canadian endocrinologist Hans Hugo Selye (1907–1982) was the first to hypothesize the fundamental division into eustress (positive stress) and distress (negative stress) based on physical responses to stressing agents of varying intensities. Negative stress or "distress" had already been the object of study for American physiologist Walter Bradford Cannon (1871–1945), whose 1929 description of the reaction to acute stress, the "fight-or-flight" response, is still used today to explain various types of reactions to stressors. This concept aimed to describe the rapid chain reaction taking place inside the body that allows it to mobilize the resources necessary to handle threatening situations.

We should clarify that in time the two *F*s of fight and flight have grown to four, or even five. The latest theories on reactions to stress have added "freeze" (a state of alertness) and "fright" (fear or tonic immobility, which includes thanatosis). To complete the picture, the fifth *F* has been identified as "faint," the loss of consciousness.

In brief, the reaction mechanisms to acute stress can be summarized thus:

1. **Freeze:** in many cases, our first reaction when presented with a threat from afar; that is, approaching but not immediate. This is also our first response to fear. To freeze in a state of alertness allows the body to process and evaluate the level of danger from a stationary position. The expression "frozen with fear" refers to this same reaction.

2. **Flight:** usually the response that follows the alert state. It is the trigger that tells the body to escape the threat in response to the perception that the danger is coming closer.

3. **Fight:** a reaction that involves no particular training in developing individual aggression. In the (real or perceived) absence of an escape route when a threat appears to come from all directions, for many the countermeasure of combat becomes the only possibility. A blind, totally uninhibited use of violence may ensue.

4. **Fright:** When other dynamic reactions seem useless, the body may react with inaction. Fallen prey to fear, the instinct to keep still is activated. This state is associated with a sort of anesthesia that numbs the senses in a final attempt not to yield fully to terror and remain conscious of what is happening.

5. **Faint:** The body is unable to handle the increasing stress, and a sudden loss of consciousness occurs. Some experts see this reaction as the body's last-ditch attempt at escape.

These reactions all have survival as their primary goal. None of them have self-destructive purposes, even if at times that may seem doubtful. In physiological terms, the classic response to a stress stimulus takes place along the amygdala-hypothalamus-pituitary-adrenal axis.

According to the American neurologist Joseph LeDoux, there are two cerebral pathways that process messages of danger from a given stimulus in the environment. The starting point, obviously, is always the sensory organs, which send the necessary information to the brain for processing. This information reaches the most "ancestral" part of the brain, the amygdala, which is responsible for activating the fear response. There are two pathways for reaching the amygdala: one goes directly from the thalamus (the "low road"), the other travels from the thalamus to the cortex and then to the amygdala (the "high road"). The thalamus-amygdala pathway is shorter, therefore the stimuli transmission system is faster. This road, unable to avail itself of the processing of information by the cerebral cortex, only supplies the amygdala with a vague, unspecific representation of the stimulus, thus triggering a purely emotional, albeit decidedly quicker, response. It's the most instinctive response, and allows us to react to a potentially dangerous stimulus before we know exactly what it is. The low road essentially triggers escape or aggression regardless of the nature of the danger. It's like seeing a garter snake on your path and beating it with a club only to realize (through processing on the brain's "high road") that it was a completely harmless animal.

Once activated, the amygdala signals the hypothalamus to send an impulse to the pituitary gland, which stimulates the adrenal glands. The adrenal medulla then secretes two powerful hormones, adrenaline and noradrenaline, while in the cortex glucocorticoid hormones are produced, in particular cortisol, stimulating the body's various systems and thus inducing the reaction (alert, attack, flight, etc.). Usually blood pressure rises, the heartbeat speeds up, and blood flows into the muscles of the limbs, which become ready to act. Digestive processes are also interrupted, while pain receptors are temporarily suppressed. This emergency response system continues the release of stress hormones in the body until the brain "deciphers" that the danger has passed. The normalization of hormonal levels is regulated by the hippocampus, a structure in the central part of the brain that assists in the formation of memory, learning, and the cognitive processes related to the emotions.

It is important to note that after the disappearance or elimination of the threat, the body does not immediately return to its normal levels from before the state of agitation: based on individual response and intensity of the stress, the necessary time period can range from twenty minutes to over an hour.

While these responses were intended for more physical, life-threatening stimuli, we deal with so many small emergencies throughout the day that trigger the same response. One North American study showed that adult individuals experience up to 50 small stress-inducing events a day. With an average recovery time of around 30 minutes for each event, it seems our bodies might be spending half the day cyclically activating and deactivating stressed states. A remarkably huge job, secretly adding to our other daily tasks.

In situations like this—much more frequent than one

might imagine—our metabolism is disrupted by a series of hormonal excesses, particularly caused by catecholamines (adrenaline and noradrenaline) and cortisol. Recently, health news has crowned cortisol "the stress hormone" par excellence, giving it an unenviable and not wholly justified fame. At the same time, medical science, shedding light once again on the difference between acute and chronic stress, is continually getting better at explaining the changes that happen because of our immune system.

It is said that the mechanisms for reacting to stress have the goal of protecting us, even saving our lives in situations of great danger. In the acute stress stage, cortisol actually supports health and allows for quicker adaptation in responding to stimuli. Its principal action is regulating the level of glycemia in the bloodstream by releasing glucose from the liver, thus also benefiting the muscles in action. It is now widely accepted that in stress situations of short duration (i.e., "acute") these mechanisms have a stimulating effect on the immune system, speeding up the resolution of an infection or the healing of a wound.

The body doesn't react to an acute stressor by generically lowering its immune defenses, but redistributes the system's cellular and humoral resources inside the body, passing through the blood to potentially exposed organs. Even the NK lymphocytes (natural killer cells, which are responsible for controlling viruses and cancers) are more active in the acute stress phase, but their functioning is heavily damaged or reduced in chronic stress conditions, just as with T lymphocytes (T-cells). It has been shown, for example, that insomnia or strongly disturbed sleep (one of the primary causes of chronic stress) not only alters the functioning of NK lymphocytes, but also interferes in immune response to vaccinations. Cortisol plays an important role in this change, precisely because its normal concentration in the body is regulated by a circadian rhythm mirroring the sleep-wake cycle.

When stimuli (even of lesser intensity) quickly follow one another over the course of the day, weeks, or months, or when the stimulus activation-deactivation mechanism gets stuck, with the amygdala continuously informing the hypothalamus of the presence of danger even when it is gone, the hippocampus is unable to regulate the adaptive response and the system ends up not functioning as it should. The result is that stress tends to become chronic, further complicating the situation.

The chronic production of cortisol translates into "low grade" tissue inflammation, with oxidative stress that can cause occasionally serious cellular damage. In conditions like these, dangerous immunodeficiencies can develop, increasing the body's susceptibility to infection from external agents. Cellular damage caused by oxidative stress can even lead to a greater risk of developing cancer.

How many times have we happened to catch a mild illness, like a little cold or stomach bug, after a burst of work-related stress or after a few nights in which we couldn't sleep because of worries or problems we encountered the previous day? These are small but important signals our body fires at us to say we need to take our foot off the gas to avoid hitting something much worse than a simple cold. In the face of these signals, rather than searching for a way to rebalance our physical and mental equilibrium, sometimes we reactivate it by turning a deaf ear and running to the pharmacy for a quick fix. In many of these situations, it would be much healthier to take a break and reflect in a beautiful natural environment that, as has been shown, allows us to expand our cognitive capacities even with complex emotional states that produce calm and serenity, promote greater relaxation, regularize our heartbeat, and modulate blood pressure.

Moreover, conditions of chronic stress can lead us to adopt behaviors and habits ranging from bad to downright unhealthy. People who are more vulnerable to daily worries (about family, work, organization, finances, etc.) tend to consume more food with a high fat content and/or sugary snacks, along with an increased likelihood of skipping meals and consuming fewer vegetables. Over time, dropping these bad habits and returning to a healthy and balanced diet becomes increasingly difficult. It's also important to remember that high levels of cortisol in the body are associated with a diet that has more animal proteins and carbohydrates on the high glycemic index (and are thus low in fiber).

If someone feels unduly troubled with a large number of problems on a daily basis, they are much less likely to engage in moderate physical activity on an occasional basis. It's clear that a sense of fatigue (physical and mental) is a constant in chronic stress: even the mere thought of going for a nice walk in the park seems overwhelming, more mentally than physically. As a result, it gets cut out of our lives entirely.

In general, we have only recently begun to consider physical exercise and, to a lesser extent, a healthy diet as behaviors that can help reduce stress in our lives, as we tend to place more value on family relationships, time management, more and better sleep, work demands, and career. The methods reported for managing stress caused by economic problems are striking: nearly 40 percent of respondents (women more than men) reported watching television for over two hours a day, and an additional 32 percent relax by spending time on the Internet. The statistics, however, do not clearly state where choosing to leave the house and take a walk in the park might stand in the rankings. From the cultural point of view, then, the most prevalent adaptive response seems to be seeking a dopamine rush—a type of "flight" that won't save anyone. Clearly, we need to find better coping mechanisms.

Scientific and Practical Interest in the Therapeutic Use of Green Space

Within the vast body of research on the interaction between natural environments and human health, the topic of "stress and immune defenses" is one of the most important.

Credit for reintroducing research into better health through green space in the contemporary context is largely due to the American researcher Roger S. Ulrich and his foundational studies conducted in the 1980s. Of particular significance is the multiyear study carried out in a hospital setting in which Ulrich showed that for patients who had undergone major surgery, those who had rooms with windows facing outdoor green space had significantly shorter recovery periods compared with those in rooms with windows overlooking urban landscapes. In fact, the former required fewer analgesics to manage postoperative pain. The study found that in similar cases the mere sight of green space (a park, garden, or nature area) could suffice to generate adaptive responses that enabled the alleviation of both physical and psychological suffering. It could also be argued that the significant reduction in recovery times was the direct result of reaching a satisfactory psychophysiological state, which surely contributed to a strong immune response, identifiable not only by the reduction in postoperative complications but also the better healing of patients' injuries. In fact, in the mid-1990s, several clinical studies demonstrated that prolonged stress can slow down the healing process for wounds and injuries because of changes at the neurological, endocrinal, and immunological levels, which were shown to activate inflammatory processes both on the epidermis and mucous membranes.

Roger Ulrich's works blazed the trail for dozens of scientific investigations seeking to explain the interaction between nature, mind, and body, and more recently, the direct connections between nature and human physiology. The results show that these relationships create mental and physical well-being on various levels, not only through the mediation of our minds.

Since the year 2000, the most investigated topics have involved nature's impact on the psyche, with a preponderance of studies on psychological well-being (primarily mental health) and the psychophysical, as well as behavioral and cognitive aspects. It is clear that problems with stress management and other modern disorders remain the scientific focus. As we shall see, this has inspired various groups to study and perfect theories and techniques for the prevention and treatment of stress-related disorders in which the role played by green space is of absolute importance.

All this has resulted in an extensive production of scientific works and theories on the therapeutic landscape, which we shall outline and discuss in the following chapter. But the disciplinary boundaries in the research on the relationship between nature and well-being have broken down. In fact, it is interdisciplinary studies that seem to contain the most in-depth research and new information.

The information in the following chapters mines these studies to supply you with the most successful techniques and applications to create healthier and more stimulating environments, in residences and workplaces alike.

We should clarify, even if it might seem obvious, that our treatment of each specific topic in the chapters ahead is by no means irrelevant to a comprehensive view of our relationship with green space. No matter which practice you may be interested in, you should always expect your actions to have effects on a physical as well as a psychological level, more or less without distinction. Ultimately, this is the foundation for the great therapeutic possibilities nature provides us.

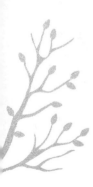

4. THE THERAPEUTIC LANDSCAPE

Of the many aspects regarding the connection between human health and green space, certainly the most studied and understood in recent decades concerns the positive effect the natural landscape has on our psychophysical well-being. How can we decipher the "therapeutic" qualities of a landscape? Are there criteria that we can use to identify one of these special landscapes?

We can try to answer this with an example. Let's go to the heart of Tuscany, in the rolling hills that extend from Siena to the peaks of Mt. Amiata. This is the border between the Crete Senesi and Val d'Orcia, a natural setting typically considered one of the most beautiful in Italy. San Giovanni d'Asso isn't the only area with the merit of being a happy mix between farmland and forest, in other words, between a tamed and a more "wild" environment. We are fully aware that talking about this place means being unfair to all the others—and there are many, not just in Italy or Europe—with similar features. But this is the place we're going to examine, right on the edge of town, on a road that leads to Asciano, the "capital" of the Crete.

Past a curve we notice an open gate, a path, and a sign alerting us to a private forest open to visitors from sunrise to sundown, where the rules are good manners and respect for other people's property, in addition to not smoking.

Faced with such an invitation, there is no choice but to enter. But this isn't just any woodland park: it's a forest-sculpture that Sheppard Craige, its creator, has decorated with art and words, mainly questions about (and to) ourselves. Philosophical, sure, but also emblematic content that reflects on the outside something that each of us could have on the inside: the Altar to Skepticism, the Center of the Universe, the Oracle of Yourself, a Place That Could Be Another . . . As its maker says, "The Bosco does not offer a meaning, but is, on the contrary, open to all interpretations." The walk starts to get interesting. A big holm oak in the middle of a clearing is at a point that feels energetically positive for our bodies: a coincidence?

The forest slopes down into a little valley casually ordered in walkways and flowerbeds filled with quotations, works of art, and symbols. At the bottom of the hill in a round pond lies a stone with the inscription "Aequus Animus," set right at the water's surface, neither over nor under, in equilibrium.

The water itself takes on a certain presence, acting as a liquid mirror for our thoughts. The rustle of the leaves accompanies the visit; other sounds fade into the background and lose importance.

Once past the various "rooms" in the forest, a road leads out into the open air, to a large area once used for agriculture but since transformed into a garden. Here the orderly trees, hedges, patterns made on the ground with stones, and walkways capture our eye and invite us to explore in a different way. Carefully laid-out seating invites us to stop and contemplate, perhaps reflect on something we have just read, like the three stones placed on the ground that say: "Not knowing, but asking," "Not asking, but thinking," "Not thinking, but doing."

In an area of approximately 35 acres, there are two natural environments that are very different from each other: a well-preserved holm oak forest and a garden governed by patterns and perspectives. In other words, an untouched natural landscape, and a manmade landscape informed by and interpreted from nature.

The serenity of the place is a constant nearly all year round, so there isn't a season in which this work of art isn't worth visiting.

The visit can't be rushed. It's almost imperative to get lost, linger, retrace your steps to see the place from another perspective, ask the Oracle of Yourself the inevitable question and then sit down to wait for the response (even if Craige warns that "answers may not be explicit"). You come out of the Bosco della Ragnaia at least a few hours after you went in with the clear sensation of having experienced something therapeutic: your relaxation is evident, your mind got "away from yourself," nature welcomed you with kindness and evoked stories that touch you personally. Sheppard Craige is an American artist who has decided to live in Italy. During a chance meeting some time ago, he responded to our enthusiasm about the therapeutic nature of his park with surprise, amusement, and indifference. Enigmatic, like certain corners of his forest.

This only proves that each of us certainly has our own sense of landscape, a personal point of view that doesn't necessarily have to coincide with a description created by someone else. It can mean something different to everyone.

Further complicating matters is the fact that most environments fit into the definition of landscape, and trying to classify or list them to establish some limits to the topic is not much help.

For our purposes, "natural landscape" means any environment, large or small, simple or complex, that is characterized by a nonnegligible presence of natural elements, from plants (hopefully alive and well) on the windowsill to the Amazon rainforest. Does this explanation seem too easy? Too generic? Only on the surface. Knowing that you have more resources than you can imagine for obtaining tangible benefits for your health should lead you to make your choices carefully rather than restrict the field by trusting prepackaged models. Even better, you can learn to express clear and above all personal preferences regarding what today we would call "nature."

It is precisely this individual vision that needs to be cultivated and developed. So instead of listing specific environments that already bear the label of "therapeutic," we'll guide you to find your own space. We won't give you a to-do list of therapeutic landscapes. There is much more that must be taken into consideration in order to find the place that makes you feel good: the search always, inevitably, begins inside you.

So let's start with ourselves, introducing the first key concept that will help you to better understand how the landscape can affect your well-being. The concept, expressed in very simple terms, is that *nature-containing landscapes have meaning for us.* Their "meaning" goes well beyond mere communication. To say that "the landscape tells us something nice or pleasant" doesn't mean that a natural environment is there to actually speak to anyone. Have you ever seen a tree calling out to a passerby? The most obvious response is "no, of course not." But that is a hasty, superficial response, because in truth some kind of communication happens. It always does.

Be aware that this communication takes a little awareness on your part. By engaging with nature, we are consciously interpreting an element of the reality around us (the landscape) as a message, or more appropriately, as something that has a certain meaning to us.

This is one of the primary reasons why nature exerts a surprising therapeutic power over human beings. When we say that a natural place provides sensations that make us feel good, we are simply drawing on our innate preference for the place where 99.5 percent of our evolutionary time has been spent (remember the genus *Homo*?): natural settings and landscapes. This inheritance is also enriched by our personal experiences with nature, which take place primarily (though not exclusively) during childhood, which in turn can influence our emotional compatibility with certain models of green space.

We must never forget our inborn biophilia. Nature is full of signs that can guide our adaptive responses toward well-being. It's just a matter of learning to recognize them better and fully grasping the meaning they have for us. In this recognition process, our rational mind initially plays an identifying role and, after that, establishes a kind of contact that, in its most effective form, would be defined as "empathy."

Therapeutic or Regenerative?

First, we should clarify our terminology, starting with "therapeutic landscape." In Western culture, the adjective "therapeutic" has become primarily associated with treating an illness or a symptom of one, but we would like to expand its sphere. In fact, the term "therapeutic landscape" is a relatively recent addition to scientific literature (introduced by Wilbert M. Gesler in 1992) in order to indicate the places or landscapes where the interactions between particular aspects of the environment, social context, and human perception create conditions favorable to a state of well-being. Thus for human beings to benefit from the therapeutic power of a natural space, they must somehow interact with it. This interaction can take all different forms. Depending on the cultural imprint of a community or an individual, a natural or seminatural place might be considered more effective than a specially "constructed" space like a garden, or the reverse. There is no reason to make distinctions or value judgments, because it is clear that there is no one place that is therapeutic for everyone.

Since nature doesn't bother to send us messages and we are the ones to interpret it and pull out perceivable meanings, it follows that at a given moment anyone could theoretically arrive at their own personal message of well-being (or suffering) in a given context.

In some cases, it is more appropriate to use the term "regenerative" than "therapeutic." Indeed, the "regenerative power of nature" effectively represents the feeling of psychophysical recuperation that comes from empathic engagement with green space. The meanings of the two terms are not perfectly interchangeable: while "therapeutic" has a more general significance, "regenerative" is used in particular for certain aspects related to the way in which the natural setting is experienced.

Identifying Disturbing Factors (in Order to Avoid Them)

It's not all flowers and sunshine: in any green space there may be underlying or intervening factors that, in various ways, disturb the visitor or even make it impossible to reach the proper state of well-being. "Disturbance" can involve all of our senses, each of which brings stimuli to our mind (the stressors we discussed previously) necessary to develop a negative experience. Let's look at a few simple examples.

Sound pollution is often at the root of failure to enjoy a natural space. No matter how aesthetically pleasing, a park afflicted with extraneous noise (traffic, construction, sirens, loud voices, shouting, and so on) inevitably loses much of its appeal. Plant barriers, like hedges or rows of trees placed along the border of the green area, generally aren't enough to combat this form of pollution. In fact, in order to lose intensity, sound waves must break against sufficiently large solid fencing or be muffled by the physical makeup of the space. The existence of nature sounds within the green space helps to mask the presence of extraneous sounds, since the human ear focuses on natural sounds over artificial ones. In the absence of effective mitigation, the disturbance could be contrasted by artificial means, like listening to music through earphones, but these are countermeasures that create a "filtered" relationship with the context and can attenuate our personal involvement with the surrounding environment (as well as others in it).

Visual disturbances are even more varied. They may concern the presence of elements discordant to the green area, such as any antennas and pylons, billboards, vehicles, buildings, and so on, as well as the existence of various forms of blight (trash, dirtiness, and dilapidated buildings). Overcrowding—another potential source of acoustic disturbance—can also keep us from appreciating green space.

Neglect or failure to maintain greenery, excessive vegetation, or unpleasant shapes of bushes and trees (deriving, for example, from inappropriate pruning) can constitute additional factors in visual disturbance. These are more difficult to mitigate than sound disturbances, and visitors may express indifference, irritation, or in any case a lack of empathy, directly as a result of the blight revealed "at first sight" of a natural place. In certain circumstances even taste can be involved in judgment (such as with leafy plants or poisonous fruit, for example), yet more often the olfactory sense conditions our perception, both from the presence of extraneous odors and rotting vegetal elements or decomposing organic substances, all stimuli that can give us the impression of visiting an unhealthy place. However, the opposite situation can also arise, in which the visitor's expectations are somehow disappointed by the lack of smells of flowers in bloom or other characteristic scents.

Another important aspect is touch, extended to the sensations that involve the entire surface of our skin. For example, in certain green spaces, thorny plants oblige us to pay attention to where we move. You can never let down your guard, so you can't relax. The same goes for certain hours of the day or periods of the year when certain environments foster the presence of bothersome insects. The sense of touch contributes a great deal to the greater or lesser emotional involvement we have with green spaces, whether natural or constructed. Walking on ground that is muddy and slippery generally doesn't facilitate relaxation, nor does lying out on a carpet of grass that's too wet or sitting on dirty or rickety benches.

Rediscovering or maintaining a certain closeness with the naturalness of a place isn't easy for many, especially those who are skeptical or find natural environments dirty to begin with. For those people, finding well-being in nature isn't as simple as visiting a park and walking barefoot on the grass. As you've seen, individual appreciation of a space can vary widely from one person to the next. When some incompatibility between aspects of the environment arises, the intrinsic significance of the place and the expectations of those who seek to visit it, the regenerative benefit of a green space is compromised.

Then what are we to do? Avoid visiting certain places? Be very picky about which spaces we visit? The answer is yes . . . and also no. Within limits, even an imperfect green space can have a positive effect on our sense of well-being; it's a question of the relationship between costs and benefits. Instead, we should avoid what disturbs us most and seek out what matches our expectations; therefore it is useful to better understand how we ourselves "function" in our surrounding environment, thanks to the explanation provided by the fascinating theory of attention restoration.

Attention Restoration Theory

The presence of negative environmental stimuli doesn't help psychic recovery from states of stress or mental fatigue, precisely because it is the stimuli themselves that generate the fatigue. Indeed, it is no easy task to keep everything that disturbs or bothers us out of our sphere of interaction (visual, auditory, tactile, and comprehensive).

According to Stephen Kaplan, researcher at the University of Michigan who developed attention restoration theory in the 1990s, human beings have two ways of focusing on their own interests, in accordance with what William James postulated in the late nineteenth century. These two modes of attention inform the way we process information in different environmental contexts.

The first type of attention is definitely involuntary: human beings home in on the information they need to process in a certain environment without making any noticeable effort. Involuntary attention kicks in when stimuli are interesting and engaging and we are able to maintain our mental reflexivity and concentration automatically, both in terms of content and active processes. In terms of energy expenditure, we could say it is a no- or low-cost mental commitment.

The more natural a place is perceived to be, the more it elicits involuntary attention. Unfortunately, not all of the stimuli that come from a given environment are interesting or engaging. In fact, it wouldn't be excessive to state that it's actually more common to encounter uninteresting and unengaging stimuli, but, regardless, they must be found and analyzed in order to be faced.

Picture a business meeting, a mental task, a difficult reading assignment, or any other thing that demands our attention in an environment that is in turn characterized by many other stimuli competing for our attention or, worse, to distract us. In these situations, human beings resort to the other form of attention, defined as direct or voluntary. This involves activating a focused interest that engages the mind on two fronts: the first to remain mentally (and physically) engaged by the information and the activities that are to be carried out; the second, more important, is to filter out all the competing stimuli, especially if they offer more appealing opportunities for relaxation or entertainment compared with the main activity going on. An inhibitory mechanism works against the competing stimuli, involving more of a mental effort and corresponding expenditure of energy.

There are individuals who are trained and efficient enough in employing direct attention that they can comfortably engage in two demanding tasks at the same time, but don't be fooled: these actions always come with a not-insignificant mental and energetic cost; they are nonetheless laborious and require a type of attention that can't be exercised efficiently for very long.

The mind, just as much as the body, needs to recover from the effort demanded by direct attention. This becomes evident in the symptoms of reduced efficiency that are seen in such cases: difficulty concentrating and memorizing, feeling tired, slowed cognitive processing, impulsivity, irritability, all symptoms that can be attributed to a state of stress.

But the brain, as we know, doesn't unplug entirely when it needs to rest. Even in the deepest sleep it remains active, albeit displaying major (and necessary) changes in activity, while in the waking hours, during everyday activities, the recovery of mental energy occurs when attention is turned toward the stimuli perceived in the moment as more interesting or pleasurable and therefore less demanding.

But which environments best facilitate this restoration of attention? Therapeutic landscapes, of course. A number of studies demonstrate the regenerative effectiveness of natural or seminatural environments compared with urban or otherwise strongly anthropized settings. As a result, whenever possible our preferences should be directed toward large gardens, parks, developed woods, meadows with trees, forests, and other similar places containing a great deal of nature.

In the absence of environments such as these, we aren't entirely doomed—we have other resources available to us, as long as we sharpen our tools for analyzing and understanding green spaces.

Kaplan's theory can come to our aid, defining the particular characteristics that an environment needs to have in order to be restorative. It should possess four properties or requirements at the same time: "being away," extent, fascination, and compatibility. These requirements constitute the first level of identification and selection of places suitable for the relief of our attention. Knowing them enables us to ask questions about what potential an environment has to meet our own personal needs. Let us provide a brief description of the four require-ments; at the end of each there are key questions useful for assessing a green space's fulfillment of the requirement.

Being Away

The expression "being away" refers to environments that ap-pear physically different and geographically distinct compared with those that belong to our everyday lives, where direct at-tention prevails. Therefore, being away indicates that percep-tion of being "somewhere else" or doing new and interesting things, physically and psychologically relaxing, creating an ad-equate distance from our daily routine. In a certain sense, it's a little bit like going on vacation.

Kaplan points out that the feeling to seek out in these places is a temporary escape from sources of mental fatigue or what is routine for us, as well as directing ourselves toward different contexts and experiencing new and engaging sensa-tions. A green space that offers a physical and emotional sepa-ration from the ordinary duties of our lives has the ability to call back up our involuntary attention.

Reflect:

- Does spending time here allow me to detach from my daily routine?

- Can I get away from the things that are occupying my attention right now?

Extent

The concept of extent can be used to describe an environment that seems sufficiently extensive and with a coherence that enables it to draw visitors' involuntary attention for long enough to allow them to explore without any particular effort. This is something much different from our everyday environments, which have borders limiting our physical and mental field of action, thus becoming the theater of our habits and repetitive stimuli that leave little room for curiosity and interest. They are almost certain not to possess "extent" requirements.

In the search for this characteristic there are not many physical dimensions of an environment that count as much as the presence of attractions: a garden structured for facilitating contemplative processes and meditation can therefore be just as effective as a park or a protected area with a high degree of naturalness. The important thing is for there to be space (i.e., extent) for our use. Put in simpler terms, they must be places that are capable of capturing and maintaining our interest.

Reflect:

- Does this place seem not to set limits (of time or of space) on my possibilities of use?

- Are there clear elements that describe and define this environment as a whole?

Fascination

The requirement that creates fascination is simpler to understand. It refers to the very appeal of the place that draws our attention, keeping it alive and constant without particular effort. Fascination, according to Kaplan, is exercised in two different ways: soft fascination and hard fascination. The first is created by environments and situations with a gentle appeal, an emotional engagement modulated by pleasurable but not overly intense stimuli, which allow for a full regenerative experience. The second presupposes intense involvement, in which the emotional part overtakes reflections and sensations but generally is less effective in restoring direct attention. Good fascination does not require direct contact with the environment. Contemplating a natural landscape from a distance, perhaps from a nice vista point, can equally occupy our attention for a sufficient amount of time to achieve the desired effects.

Reflect:

• Can this place be defined as appealing?

• Do I feel absorbed by this scene?

Compatibility

The last requirement, compatibility, indicates an environment's ability to support both our intentions and our expectations. The correspondence between individual demand and the particulars of the environment should be such that it avoids, for example, the emergence of states of anxiety, disappointment, boredom, or irritation. If an individual looking for solace in green space is burdened by mental and physical fatigue, they should search for a place of peace and calm, and should avoid environments that provide opportunities for movement, exercise, and exploration, like green areas with playground equipment, running trails, or open space for collective use. Climbing a mountain obviously wouldn't be so "compatible."

Reflect:

• Does being in this place coincide with my interests at this moment?

• Does this environment offer the opportunities for fun and relaxation that I'm looking for?

These questions should be taken as examples; they could be replaced with others that achieve the same purpose. To better digest their significance, it would be a good idea to practice these requirements on a regular basis, especially trying to describe a natural environment that seems to have regenerative qualities, similar to our discussion of the Bosco della Ragnaia at the beginning of this chapter.

It should also be said that fulfilling all of Kaplan's requirements may not always be easy. A place considered ideal might not be very close by, leading us to look into other possibilities and alternatives. This is why recognizing the characteristics of an environment and its ability to meet our expectations is always a useful exercise.

Toward Making Conscious Choices

There is actually a lot of information available to us for finding, choosing, or even imagining one or more landscapes we could use for psychophysical recuperation, especially for chronic stress. Before going into detail, let's briefly review the most important aspects you should keep in mind.

The first has to do with the concept of biophilia. We are "biological individuals," meant to live in contact with nature. Although we constantly adopt controlled and formal behaviors and habits, when we find ourselves in natural environments we tend to act in a much more instinctive way, expressing our preferences and broadly yielding to our unconscious reflexes. This is confirmed by the environmental stimuli that generate responses of alert or make us instantly more cautious, such as dark places, precipices, wild animals, and so forth. However, we are equally quick to relax in the presence or sight of open places, calm but not static, with the right ratio of light to shadow, and enough vegetation to allow for surveillance and interpretation of the environment.

Models of green space that resemble the landscape of the savanna at least somewhat provide the fastest adaptive response of recovery from stress. In these environments, humans find familiarity with a model of place that represented their home for a very long time. Our bodies automatically relax, and the sensation is even more obvious for those of us who are predisposed to suffer more from states of stress. This model of landscape is an archetype we have carried inside us for millennia. But it is not the only one.

The second aspect is quantitative. We could say that the more nature there is, the better it is for our well-being, even if the quality of the nature does matter a great deal. Living in proximity to large green areas extends our life and lowers the risk of contracting certain illnesses, as several studies and surveys conducted on significant swaths of the population show. How effective the action of nature will be often depends on how long we spend in it and the "dose" we take of it, as we will see farther on. This is a recurring rule not to be forgotten or underestimated.

The third aspect involves the trust with which we approach natural spaces. We ought to come into contact with these environments without putting up filters, freeing ourselves from certain mind-sets and prejudices about supposed dangers, opening ourselves up—if and when possible—to socialization. Sometimes it doesn't take much, even less than you might think.

Those with experience hiking, for example, find it normal to greet the people they meet on their path. Occasionally they stop to chat with a stranger for the sole purpose of being friendly, whereas in a more anthropized place this exchange is far less likely to happen. In a big city, it can be almost impossible.

The level of interaction one might find comfortable in a certain environment varies. The stimuli resulting from a work or social context full of tasks and responsibilities may be overwhelming for someone under stress. Too much involvement with that sort of environment can be unsustainable.

Yet in a more natural space we can experience a degree of involvement that is more compatible with our psychophysical state. Interacting with animals, for example, certainly doesn't require the commitment required of most work relationships (unless they involve a hungry crocodile, of course). Plants have even fewer demands than animals, thus they make it possible to take a more relaxed approach, and the inanimate components of a landscape, like a pond, rock, or statue, ask even less—they let themselves be observed without expecting anything. They don't even oblige you to think about the cycle of life, unlike plants, through the stages of their development. A "thoughtfully engaged" relationship with a natural environment enables you to recover with ease, without imposition, your personal capacity for self-control and action, as well as cognitive and decision-making abilities. It gives us the space to reconnect with ourselves.

Moreover, our relationships with others become more manageable and spontaneously oriented toward cooperation, rather than comparison and competition. This comprehensive recuperation can influence our physiology—on the level of all our systems, including the immune system—and therefore improve our general quality of life.

Experiencing our capacity for engagement (or disengagement) with a place or a situation perceived as manageable can be very healthy; it also fulfills the requirement of "being away" for the restoration of direct attention.

Our Mental Energies: A Pyramid to Climb

More or less during the years in which Stephen Kaplan was perfecting attention restoration theory, in the landscape planning department at the Swedish University of Agricultural Sciences in Alnarp, researchers led by Professor Patrik Grahn investigated personal capabilities of involvement and participation in experiences with nature.

In 1991, Grahn developed a model called the visitor's mental power, which connected the state of an individual's mental energy with their ability to interact with an environment, organized in a pyramid with four levels.

The lowest level, the one with the widest base, is occupied by subjects with few mentally energetic resources (people who are ill, suffering, or severely stressed), who can only socially interact in environments that require modest instances of involvement, whether physical or mental.

The base of the pyramid represents individual demand well. These people need a fairly large amount of individual (i.e., not shared) space and structurally simple environments, easy to interpret, that facilitate an inner engagement and also allow for simple activities at the physical level, like sitting or walking in calm places away from sources of disturbance.

The next level includes people who are mentally active, capable of putting their impressions and thoughts in order, but who aren't prepared to consider new ideas or reflections suggested by others or to share. It isn't so much solitude that these people seek as less involvement with what is outside the self. The quota of individual space required is not as large as at the first level: the field of observation can also include other people who are active or in motion, but proper distance must be maintained. A natural environment can offer more interest. For example, noticing the natural plant cycle (observing sprouts, fruits, the falling of leaves, etc.) is not unwelcome, and contemplation can also leave room for curiosity.

The third level of the pyramid contains the individuals who have restored their physical health and a good part of their mental health and can participate emotionally in the environment they are immersed in. The quota of individual space is lower and shared with others who have a similar level of mental energy; they can therefore manage relations with their neighbors and engage in conversation without any antisocial behavior arising. Even participating in the natural environment becomes more intense and can include various activities, such as exploring an unknown place or making empathic contact with plants and animals.

The very top of the pyramid holds all the people who aim for active participation and relate to others in an engaging manner. The quota of individual space needed in this case is minimal and largely shared with the group. They can attempt more challenging activities, even at the physical level, and their environmental involvement is characterized by creativity and confidence (they often act as leaders).

Grahn's model allows us to better understand how our ability to relate to a given environment changes, just as our mental energies vary. This can inform the quality and quantity of green space that we need to help us get over feelings of stress or psychophysical fatigue, or just to distract us from a laborious task.

In order to find the most restorative space, you must ask yourself which level of the pyramid best fits your current situation.

The Search for "Our" Therapeutic Landscape

The experience of searching for the "ideal" characteristics of a landscape chosen for our well-being is almost as important as the experience of being in it. Both the rational-cultural part of us and the more instinctive part contribute more or less equally in finding it. With our more rational mind, we can make use of all the experience and information we have thus far acquired to make a decision, whereas our subconscious will tap into our instinctive reactions in response to a particular natural setting.

To start, let's look at some practical aspects. The first is accessibility, defined both in terms of our distance from the green space and the possibility of exploring the place safely (compatibility). The importance of how far away a place is should not be underestimated—recent studies have shown that how frequently a green space is visited (a park or urban forest, in most cases) and the time spent in it are inversely proportional to the location's distance from our residence or workplace. It may seem hard to believe, but notable differences have been found in the type and frequency of visits even with distances of a few dozen feet. The threshold of 1,000 feet from a green space seems to be what marks the shift from regular to occasional visits, with the necessary corrections and variations based on various geographical and climatic factors. Consider that 1,000 feet is the average distance an adult can cover in 5 to 6 minutes in an urban setting.

Lack of time is the most common circumstance keeping us from visiting green space. This was the answer given by over

60 percent of interviewees on a survey conducted on a sample of 953 residents of Sweden's major cities. The second reason was distance from the home. These reasons are applicable not just to people in the Scandinavian countries but to all Western societies.

If we find a green space that meets our environmental expectations but is found at a distance of several miles from our home or place of work, we will need more time and stronger reasons to visit it with any regularity. Otherwise we risk going only when something is wrong or we're so stressed we go to nature as a last resort. Yet it is evident that occasional use of green spaces for therapeutic purposes generally produces "occasional," that is, negligible, results. As we have already said, how effective natural environments are in providing us with psychophysical benefits is often the product of a time- and dose-dependent mechanism. The dose is represented by how often we visit a green space and how long we stay each time. It may be advisable, therefore, to choose more than one place to visit, assigning each different values and aims in consideration of what each has to offer. We should keep in mind the parameter of reaching this space in 5 to 6 minutes by walking and try not to minimize its importance.

For those who live in the city and don't have a park in the immediate vicinity, daily empathic contact may be fulfilled with a plant-filled terrace or backyard, as long as these spaces have enough meaning to inspire our individual appreciation. It is indeed very unlikely, impossible even, for a garden left untended and dominated by tall weeds to elicit any sort of soft fascination with notable therapeutic power. Even in wilder natural environments, there is a characteristic order with its own coherence (extent) that is able to give people a strong sense of harmony.

A garden, therefore, must be looked after, or it cannot carry out its functions. Gardens follow a personal archetype and should be treated as an extension of our house toward the outside world, as if it were an additional room. Like all the other rooms, it indeed has a floor (the lawn, flowerbeds, and walkways, for example), walls (hedges, fencing, or an actual wall), and a ceiling (the treetops, if not the sky itself). Since the era of the Mesopotamian civilizations, gardens have broadly maintained this archetypal structure, a structure that works best when we tend it in a way that activates our well-being. It was not happenstance that the first hospitals erected in the Middle Ages in monastery complexes always overlooked a garden, a *hortus conclusus*. These were therapeutic spaces that allowed the ill and convalescent to benefit from an airy, sunny environment protected from the elements, to ensure them a faster recovery from the illness or trauma they had suffered.

As they become increasingly far from our homes, natural environments must be more carefully sought out, and must correspond as closely as possible to the four fundamental requirements described by Kaplan. In fact, the appeal of a more natural place filled with meaning, compared with a small urban green space, can produce the necessary motivation for healthier and more consistent visits.

It is also important to keep track of the levels of use that each green space has to offer. There are three levels: visual, presence, and activity. These relate not only to the intrinsic and structural characteristics of a place but also to our mental energies (as you've seen in the pyramid structure of the visitor's mental power). In general, environments that offer all these opportunities are the ones that are most appreciated by visitors.

Visual

The level of visual use is applicable to all nature-containing environments, from balconies with plants to dense forests. Visual use affects our well-being particularly through soft fascination, often in a very powerful way. Seeing the plants on our terrace grow and bloom is in itself a form of restoration of direct attention, which for a few satisfying minutes can take us away from our daily worries.

Presence

We can also take a more active role in restoring direct attention by learning to use our involuntary attention more often. As we walk through the city, or even in a rural environment, how often do we stop to look at a tree, any tree? How many times have we appreciated its shape, colors, stature, aesthetic, its overall harmony? We should set out to do so, knowing that every interested and conscious look is a real contribution to restoring our direct attention, and therefore a small step toward recuperating our mental energy. Spending time in a natural context is a human need that is truly rich with meaning. It is a demonstration of our sense of belonging to the environment, which is in turn nourished by our instincts and all the experiences we have had with nature. Our presence in nature prompts us to contemplation and reflection, but it also stimulates curiosity and the desire to understand the significance and coherence of a place.

When you feel a pull to be present, the restorative properties of a space are likely already working on you. The need to be "in" the landscape also signals the existence of the desire to heal: it is the message we send ourselves by favorably interpreting the signs of nature.

Activity

Activities are at the core of many therapeutic practices involving green space. Horticultural therapy is a prime example. In order to practice it, you don't need to have an actual garden, just a few pots on a balcony, a little imagination, and a desire to learn how to plant. But even everyday physical activities practiced in nature are essential for our health. Furthermore, it has been widely demonstrated that they not only improve our cognitive performance but also create less of a sense of fatigue than we would have from the same activity carried out indoors. A work meeting? Brainstorming session? It would definitely be worthwhile to organize these activities in view or in the presence of a pleasant natural environment. Try taking a walk in the park with a colleague instead of having lunch indoors. When we are in contact with nature or performing physical activity outside, our involuntary attention works in the background, lowering the amount of energy needed to maintain direct attention and not get distracted. Taking part in activities outdoors, in a green space, thus leads us to more "sustainable" energy consumption.

Observing, being present, and acting are processes commensurate with our mental and physical energies. Like a tailor-made dress, each can be the most apt and opportune for a certain moment in our search for well-being. When we choose "our" therapeutic landscape, we must take into account what the landscape itself communicates to us, or the meaning it evokes in us. You'll instinctively be able to grasp that message. Participation takes place at the sensory level: colors, shapes, sense of space, sounds, smells, tastes—why not? Don't we want to taste a wild fruit or an edible flower?—tactile sensations, and intuition.

Our sixth sense, in fact, is intuition. Keep in mind that some of our choices will be intuitive and yet conditioned by models, or, rather, by archetypes that we carry with us. It would be useful to recall some of the more important ones.

If we ask a child to draw a tree, in most cases they will represent it with a wide, round top and a fairly short trunk; this is the classic form that prevails in popular culture among the images of trees deemed "beautiful." The description-type is a relatively thick treetop with a trunk branching out at a not excessive distance from the ground. Several researchers have investigated this preference, finding that the shape of the acacias typical of the African savanna is privileged over those of oaks, pines, palms, or eucalypti. Column and cone shapes are generally less preferable than more expansive shapes. The "ideal" figure of the tree is thus one of the archetypes that we discussed earlier. Other preferences include open places, with a position from which we can oversee the entire scene, and settings that include the presence of water.

LANDSCAPE ARCHETYPES

Further studies have shown that the environment also intervenes in our imaginary model of a tree. When we picture trees in a natural context, we identify them with the shape of the African acacia. If we imagine them in an urban setting, there is more freedom of choice of the models themselves (within the limits of the climate of the particular location). For example, in countries with a Mediterranean climate, palm trees are also appreciated in urban contexts, whereas in northern countries pines are preferred. Yet as we imagine farther away from the city, the portrait of the shape-type goes back to being the expansive foliage and trunk that branches out quickly. The archetype therefore emerges in full force as soon as we start to connect—even just mentally—with a more natural setting.

It is useful to keep these preferences in mind when we analyze the components of a landscape, because certain plant forms communicate with us better than others do. Another archetype that affects our preferences for a place is the "panorama." Humans systematically prefer places from which they can oversee the entire scene. A panoramic point increases our sense of safety, especially if we are in a location with protection behind us (sometimes even overhead). This is an image-model that should be applied, when possible, to dwellings. Practitioners of feng shui know this archetype, considered optimal for the circulation of energies both outside and inside a home.

A landscape has a greater chance of improving our well-being if it offers many dominant positions to choose from for surveillance. When the topography of a place doesn't allow us to find an elevated position with sufficient surveillance capability, our preference goes toward environments where the vegetation is not dense and there are no obstacles to visual (or physical) exploration.

Water has a very powerful significance at the unconscious level and invariably represents life sustenance. Evolutionary theory explains the reasons why a natural setting endowed with a significant presence of water (whether a stream, river, lake, or seashore) is so preferential. The first human communities formed in places with abundant water. Rift Valley, considered the cradle of the genus *Homo,* is an extensive geographic trench in East-Central Africa dotted with small and large lakes fed by numerous freshwater streams. It is plausible that our genetic imprint related to preference for places with lots of water comes from there.

The water component of our therapeutic landscape is therefore important. Often it isn't even necessary to see it. It can be enough just to hear the sound of a stream running over rocks or ocean waves crashing softly on the shore, nature sounds that induce relaxation and serenity (as various clinical trials have shown as well).

The simultaneous presence of simple archetypes variously distributed throughout the landscape can also give rise to more complex archetypal models, which at first glance can seem difficult to interpret and appreciate. In reality, humans have proven to have innate resources when it comes to understanding the significance of a landscape, whether natural or constructed (like a park or a garden).

The aforementioned Scandinavian researchers who refer to Patrik Grahn and Ulrika K. Stigsdotter have tried to decipher these complex archetypes. In 2001, they identified eight descriptive characteristics deriving from the same number of models of garden that can possibly be defined as "therapeutic." The studies of these models in different applicable contexts (including China) allowed them to determine that correlations existed between the traits of a landscape and the preferences expressed by the individuals who took part in the survey, who were visitors of parks and other natural spaces. We could say that these traits "communicated" directly with the visitor, who in turn could interpret the sensations received by expressing a clear preference. For example, the model-archetypes represented by calm, spacious, lush, or rich characteristics, perhaps containing cultural and artistic elements, were the landscapes that attracted individuals with uncertain health. Open spaces with dynamic elements that encouraged exploration, play, or entertainment were generally appreciated by less-stressed individuals who were inclined toward group activities or curious about what others were doing.

This means that human beings are able to interpret even complex signs of nature, reflexively understanding how to choose the environments most suited to their requirements for well-being.

We should thus trust in our abilities to interpret the meaning of a place. We already have the tools at our disposal:

- analysis and assessment of factors of sensory disturbance

- the necessary requisites for restoring attention as described by Kaplan (being away, extent, fascination, compatibility)

- analysis of our mental energies and our degree of involvement in a certain environment (in terms of the visual, presence, and activity)

- assessment of our distance from green space and the time we can devote to it

- the presence and perception of archetypes that trigger our preferences (the "savanna" model of open space, the "room" model for gardens, the form of vegetation, the view, the presence of water, and so on)

Now the only thing left is to enthusiastically set off on our search.

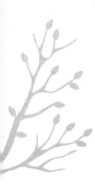

5. FOREST BATHING

Some of the most concrete evidence in support of the therapeutic abilities of green space has come in recent years from research on the monoterpenes emitted by plants. It's a brand-new perspective that could demolish once and for all the widespread (and mostly misinformed) opinion that nature acts in a way that is beneficial to humankind only through a mechanism activated or mediated by the brain. While it is very true that the human mind makes an essential contribution in regulating many physiological processes influenced by the environment, there is a measurable benefit to the immune system from forest bathing, regardless of how the person feels about nature. If the forest area is sufficiently rich in monoterpenes, even someone who isn't motivated to seek nature's benefits will receive regular help for their immune systems.

Monoterpenes have significant importance for human

health. To understand it better, we'll begin by presenting the agents of this biochemical action.

A Well-Nourished Group of Biomolecules

Monoterpenes compose a fairly large group of molecules of organic origin that are part of the larger family of terpenes (or terpenoids). Typically they are characterized by a "skeleton" of ten carbon atoms, a relatively simple structure. Their molecular weight is fairly low, which contributes to their volatility, that is, their tendency to pass from an aeriform or gaseous state in ordinary pressure conditions and atmospheric temperature.

Monoterpenes are quite common in nature, as they are produced by many plants (as well as by fungi, bacteria, and certain insects, albeit to a lesser extent) and are the typical components of resins, essential oils, and more. Rarely does a plant species produce only one type of monoterpene. Often there is one predominant molecule in a mixture that forms the essential oil, but it is even more common for there to be a composition with multiple predominant molecules. Their biological effect derives from the overall combination of substances (called a phytocomplex) rather than one individual component, so that even a terpene contained in trace amounts or a minimal quantity can noticeably alter both the sensory characteristics and the very biological properties of the essential oil. Lemon scent is a case in point. The primary monoterpene is limonene, which makes up about 70 percent of the essential oil, but the characteristic aroma is derived from citral, which represents less than 5 percent of all fragrances.

Monoterpenes are the principal sources of the particular scents of leaves, flowers, and other parts of plant organisms. Many scents used in the food industry or in perfume are in fact derived from monoterpenes, or in any case from natural terpenoids. The chemical name sometimes makes it easy to associate the terpenoid with the typical plant it comes from: limonene, alpha- and beta-pinene, eucalyptol, menthol, geraniol, camphor . . .

However, the same type of monoterpene can be produced by different plants: what is interesting is its percentage in the composition of the typical essential oil of a species. The approximately thousand monoterpenes we know of in the plant world are produced by about fifty botanical families, most prominently the Labiatae (or Lamiaceae: sage, mint, rosemary, lavender, etc.) and the Rutaceae (rue or citrus). But there are other families as well, represented mostly by tree species, which are equally worthy of interest. Furthermore, species that produce many fragrances and others that produce hardly any can coexist within the same botanical family.

Essential oils have been known to humans for thousands of years and their medicinal use is extremely widespread across all latitudes, though there are other uses as well. Pyrethrins, for example, are some of the most potent natural insecticides. Virtually harmless to mammals, they are a deadly poison for an insect's nervous system, causing paralysis within seconds of contact. The pyrethrin extracted from the Asteraceae family is used as an insecticide in farming and home environments precisely due to its low toxicity for humans and its quick decomposition in the environment.

The biological effect of monoterpenes on humans is known in a smaller number of substances compared with the number that have been identified in nature. Generally the action of the phytocomplex, or essential oil, is studied, rather than the individual molecule. Essential oils have many biological properties and a remarkable affinity with the lipid fraction of human cell membranes, so they are absorbed fairly easily through the skin or mucous membranes. This aspect has great relevance for those who visit a forest with the aim of boosting their immune defenses.

The olfactory duct is the most direct way to reach the receptors of the central nervous system. This is why the effects of inhalation are so rapid. The natural action of monoterpenes is also expressed at the cerebral level, like stimulants or sedatives, anxiolytics and antidepressants, with positive effects on both memory and cognitive processes, as well as mood.

Among the other effects of monoterpenes on the human body, the following are especially worthy of note:

- **stimulation of the mucous glands in the airways** (as expectorant or decongestant)

- **stimulation of the gastric glands** (digestive agent)

- **rubefacient and counterirritant or causes warming of the skin** (typical of camphor and eucalyptus)

- **antiseptic action** (thymol)

- **antispasmodic** (menthol) and analgesic action

Recent research in the biomedical field has shown a protective action in terms of cancer prevention, especially the essential oils *Nigella sativa* (black caraway), *Cuminum cyminum* (common cumin), *Papaver somniferum* (opium poppy), and *Ocimum sanctum* (holy basil). Other studies report the existence of liver-protecting properties. And we can't forget stimulation of the immune system, which we will return to frequently.

While essential oils are generally quite well known for their properties in human use, the role (or roles) they have in the lives of plants is less clear. We know that they fulfill various metabolic functions, some of which are not too dissimilar from those observed in human beings. We must suppose, however, that these substances are quite important for the plants, since their spread in the atmosphere as volatile compounds constitutes a real loss of organic carbon deriving from photosynthesis. Why else would a plant deprive itself of a substance that isn't just a waste product of the metabolic process?

It has been observed that under conditions of stress some plants release more monoterpenes than normal. Even isoprene, the basic molecule of these chemical compounds, can amount to nearly 40 percent of all organic carbon losses of the entire plant, whereas in normal conditions its emission into the atmosphere never surpasses 2 percent. Plants seem to produce isoprene and monoterpenes to protect themselves from environmental stress, since those molecules perform specific antioxidant and/or thermoprotective functions. This protection also extends to biotic stress agents, such as certain animal parasites, especially insects. Monoterpenes, or, rather, essential oils, in certain cases act as repellents to potential pests and potential "consumers," such as many herbivorous animals.

However, plant intelligence isn't limited to just that; some plants emanate scents to attract predators of the insects that could parasitize them. Essentially, they try to surround themselves with potential (and unknowing) outside defenders. Moreover, since monoterpenes work fairly well as chemical "messengers," many higher plants have developed their scent production further to attract pollinators, and not only from the insect class, but also bats and certain birds, such as hummingbirds.

Finally, it is interesting to consider where these substances are produced and where they accumulate (when they do) within plant structures. Biochemical synthesis takes place primarily in the aerial part of a plant, especially the leaves, but also in the young branches, the flowers, the fruit, and to a lesser extent at the base of the stem or wooden parts. They can also be found in bark, as in the Ceylon cinnamon tree. Roots may also be able to produce monoterpenes, thus contributing to the amount of emissions from the ground. Some plants are able to store these products in specialized structures such as resin ducts (canals inside leaves and wood that contain resins), or in glands, glandular hairs, vesicles, and analogous anatomical formations. Others lack "storage" structures, so they release monoterpenes into the atmosphere as soon as they are produced. Many deciduous trees have this characteristic, whereas conifers are able to accumulate large amounts of monoterpenes in their resin ducts. It's helpful to keep this in mind when planning for "immersion" activities in the woods, but there are more aspects that should be taken into consideration.

We have already noted that certain plant species produce

more monoterpenes than others. However, differences exist not only between very different species; they can be quite marked even between related trees. For example, the American beech (*Fagus grandifolia*) and the European beech (*Fagus sylvatica*) are two forest species that occupy similar habitats in their respective continents of the Northern Hemisphere, but the monoterpene emission rate of the American species is significantly lower than that of the European species.

The climate of an environment and geographical exposure can cause differences in emissions even within the same species, or even the same plant. Typically, leaves that are most exposed to light produce more monoterpenes than those that are located in the shade, even within a single tree. Furthermore, seasonal progression has a significant influence on plant production of monoterpenes. It is clear that all broadleaved deciduous species such as beech (*Fagus sylvatica*) or red maple (*Acer rubrum*) produce the most at the beginning of summer, when their leaf mass is more extensive, yet only negligible amounts in winter. But there are also important differences within evergreen species. For example, a typical Mediterranean oak, the holm (*Quercus ilex*), is more active in late spring and early fall. In general, with species that can accumulate essential oils in specific structures of their foliage, such as conifers, their monoterpene emission is mainly linked to heat (therefore, higher in summer than in winter, and in late morning to early afternoon than at night).

Plants without accumulation structures, such as many deciduous trees, produce and emit monoterpenes depending on both air temperature and amount of light, namely, environmental factors that influence photosynthesis, the process underlying the biosynthesis for all organic substances constituting plant structures. What does all this information have to do with our health? Let's start with the country where the most innovative research has been conducted: Japan.

In the East, It's Known as Shinrin-Yoku

Japan is about two-thirds covered in woods and forests, and thus it is a very green country. The Japanese define "forest" as a formation of plants in which trees cover at least 30 percent of the ground, and trees must reach a minimum height of 16 feet. The minimum surface area of each individual formation must be at least 32,000 square feet and the width must be over 65 feet. This definition is quite similar to what is used in other countries, with some differences in the breadth and extent of land cover.

As in all the major Eastern civilizations, the relationship between humans and nature is very important in Japan. There has been a relatively recent resurgence of interest in environmental issues, but the Japanese's cultural and physical bonds with nature have very ancient origins, and are also expressed in widespread personal health practices. Because of these strong bonds, and inspired by traditional practices conducted in green space in the pursuit of psychophysical well-being, in 1982 the Japanese forest service inaugurated shinrin-yoku, which is a full-immersion journey into the forest atmosphere. In English, this term was translated as "forest bathing trip," or simply "forest bathing," which we can define as entering and "soaking up" a forest environment. The reasons behind this initiative were based on the then-current knowledge about the medicinal properties of natural environments, though more from popular culture than direct scientific research. Yet shinrin-yoku was already so well known that the government campaign was an effortless success, which contributed to the spread of the practice throughout the country.

Twenty years later, likely due to the worldwide growth of scientific publications in the field, a group of Japanese researchers decided to conduct a more in-depth study on the effects of forest baths on human health. They came up with this slightly technical definition: "a visit to a public forest for relaxation and recreation during which you inhale aromas called phytoncides (wood essential oil), volatile organic compounds deriving from trees such as alpha-pinene and limonene." This refers to the release in the atmosphere of plant-produced monoterpenes, which were breathed in by visitors like a sort of natural aromatherapy session.

This early research was primarily oriented toward the stress-relieving action of shinrin-yoku. Its effects on human physiology were easily measurable, such as lowered cortisol in the saliva and lower amount of hemoglobin in the blood flowing to the prefrontal cortex of the brain. Shinrin-yoku was then compared with analogous sessions of walking and resting in an urban area, and the differences between groups in the experiment were significant: forest bathing produced a clearly relaxing effect that could be detected in the hormones as indicated above, while the city sessions did not.

In the same time frame, similar research was conducted in a very old deciduous forest in the Yamagata Prefecture, broadening the field of observed effects that the practice has on human physiology: blood pressure, pulse, and regularity of heart rate, and the concentration of cortisol and immunoglobulin A in the saliva. In addition, participants filled out a questionnaire to evaluate their subjective responses to the shinrin-yoku experience. Answers demonstrated the positive outcome of reducing typical symptoms of stress and the resulting favorable repercussions on the body.

No surprise there, we might say. This is a classic example of the therapeutic landscape we discussed in the previous chapter, which heals by restoring direct attention, fostering spontaneous relaxation, and reducing stimuli on the amygdala-hypothalamus-pituitary-adrenal axis.

The brain, decoding a positive message from the environment, produces an adaptive response that leads to a condition of greater psychophysical well-being that has been measured in numerous biomedical studies conducted in various parts of the world over the last twenty-five years. One doctor in Japan, the previously mentioned Qing Li from the Department of Hygiene and Public Health at Nippon Medical School in Tokyo, and his colleagues decided to investigate the effect on the immune system triggered by monoterpenes emitted in the forests where shinrin-yoku was practiced. In 2006, the results of the laboratory investigations conducted to assess the effect of the essential oils from two very common conifers in Japan (*Chamaecyparis obtusa* and *Cryptomeria japonica*) on the activity level of particular human lymphocytes were published in the journal *Immunopharmacology and Immunotoxicology*. The immune system cells chosen for the lab test consisted of a line of natural killer lymphocytes (NK-92MI) that intervene in the control of viruses and neoplastic cells.

These cells were kept in precise environmental conditions (i.e., in reproducible circumstances), with different concentrations of essential oils from the two conifers. The effective contact dose was very low: just 0.1 milligrams of essential oil per kilogram of culture medium. The effective contact time was shown to be at least 120 hours; after that, there was a notable increase in the metabolic activity of the NK lymphocyte cultures and intense multiplication, a clear sign of the positive stimulus provided by the phytocomplex. As part of the same laboratory test, it was further noted that pretreatment with the same dose of essential oils improved the resistance of NK lymphocytes to a toxic solution containing a known pesticide. The stimulus triggered by the essential oils clearly depended on the dose and duration of contact. Once the treatment dropped below a certain concentration and a certain amount of time, positive activities were not detected. This experiment showed the direct effect of essential oils on human immune function, in the total absence of activation or regulation by the brain. It was a sensational discovery, which Dr. Li reinforced with further studies in the field (or rather, the forest) seeking to demonstrate the effectiveness of shinrin-yoku in producing direct benefits to the immune system.

Field experiments, which were repeated for several years from 2005 on, involved groups of people of both sexes and between the ages of 25 and 55, in good health, who followed a trip protocol for a visit of three days and two nights in forest areas in three different Japanese prefectures. The protocol was the following: each day of the visit required a walk of at least two hours through the woods, which was doubled (two hours in the morning and two hours in the afternoon) on the second day. Participants could stop and rest at any time, but were asked to travel an average of at least 2.5 kilometers per walk. The same program was followed by a control group, but on a tour of Nagoya, a city with artistic/historical attractions. None of the selected participants had practiced shinrin-yoku in the three months prior to the experiment. Each morning the participants had to provide blood and urine samples to determine:

- the number of white blood cells, number and activity of natural killer lymphocytes (NK), number of T lymphocytes, and amount of intracellular anticancer proteins in the blood;

- the concentration of adrenaline and noradrenaline in the urine, since these are stress hormones and partly responsible for reducing NK lymphocyte activity.

The first sample was taken a few days before the start of the experiment on a regular weekday and then repeated on all three days of the practice, then one week after and one month after. Over the course of the experiment, the concentration of monoterpenes in the air was also measured in various points of the forest.

The results of the analyses showed a significant increase in the number (over 40 percent, going as high as 50) and activity level of NK lymphocytes even after the second day's visit, with a significant increase in the amount of anticancer proteins within the cells of peripheral blood lymphocytes. Furthermore, the levels of adrenaline and noradrenaline in the urine had gone down as soon as the first day's visit. In the control group, composed of subjects involved in the tourist trip, no significant variations in the number and activity of lymphocytes, nor in the urinary level of stress hormones, were found. A very interesting aspect of the experiment was how long the benefits to the immune system lasted. In fact, one week after the forest trip, the activity and number of NK lymphocytes remained high and only after thirty days did blood tests indicate a slight decline. In practice, the immune system received a boost with effects that lasted over a month. They concluded that regular visits to forest areas with a significant production of monoterpenes in accordance with the protocol laid out by the Japanese researchers helps to keep the immune defenses high.

These experiments carried out in Japan led the researchers to conclude that the practice of shinrin-yoku can increase the activity level of NK lymphocytes and the intracellular content of anticancer proteins—so-called forest bathings can thus have a preventive effect on carcinogenesis and the development of tumors. Qing Li's studies have been reported and cited in dozens of subsequent works of research, both experimental and in reviews, demonstrating the scientific world's growing interest in these recent discoveries.

In the West, It's Known as Forest Bathing

The results of these experiments quickly spread around the world, finding the biggest foothold in the United States, where the practice has been called forest bathing. In 2015, Spafinder Wellness UK Ltd., the world's leading media, marketing, and gift company in the wellness industry, placed forest bathing in first place of the "global top ten" trends among spa and wellness center visitors. In the same period, over a hundred studies on the health impact of forest bathing and similar practices appeared in the PubMed research database. Today, there are countless websites promoting various ways of practicing forest bathing, and the topic seems to be exhaustively covered.

That said, to achieve real results, you'll need a little more background. Which forests can produce monoterpenes in adequate amounts to provide beneficial effects on our immune system? This simple question may be enough to indicate that the subject is anything but exhausted. Let us try to fill in these essential information gaps.

The Japanese researchers, during the experiments they conducted in the forest, measured the concentration of phytoncides in the air. The values calculated the principal monoterpenes in the tree species prevalent in the forests where the studies were done: alpha- and beta-pinene, camphene, tricyclene, limonene, isoprene, and so on. The quantities detected were below one hundred, a few hundred at most, nanograms (i.e., fractions of micrograms) per cubic meter of air. In such concentrations, a particular essential oil is not perceptible at the olfactory level. For example, the smell of coniferous wood is largely caused by L-limonene and alpha-pinene, whose threshold of perception for humans is a few milligrams per cubic meter of air: one milligram corresponds to a thousand micrograms. All that can be recognized is simply the typical scent of the forest, composed of smells from soil and plants, especially when there are ideal temperature conditions and relative humidity in the air. Our sense of smell, therefore, can't guide us very effectively in searching for the best source of monoterpenes—humans aren't bloodhounds.

Moreover, it is well known that the Japanese conifers *Cryptomeria japonica* and *Chamaecyparis obtusa* are certainly not the only species capable of emitting monoterpenes (fortunately so!). It is thus necessary to know which other trees can produce the most effective atmospheric concentrations for our immune systems.

It is worth mentioning that the effect of the substances contained in essential oils on human lymphocytes follows a dose- and time-dependent mechanism. Regarding exposure time, we have fairly precise information. Japanese protocols indicate that about ten hours over three days is sufficient, with visits in the forest of at least two hours for each visit, taking into account the possible variability in individual responses to these kinds of biochemical stimuli. Even with a lack of time, a single visit of at least three to four hours can bring about the first (partial) positive effects: measurements taken after the first day of walking in the woods showed a noticeable decrease in the levels of adrenaline and noradrenaline in the body. And what about the most effective dose—how can we pace ourselves?

Fortunately, a specific branch of bioclimatology studies the relationships between volatile organic compounds (called VOCs, which also include monoterpenes) and the gases responsible for the greenhouse effect to identify the most suitable potential species for forest bathing. Vegetation in the Northern Hemisphere (especially Europe and North America) has been—and continues to be—widely studied by bioclimatologists for the role it plays in the regulation of greenhouse gases at the level of the continental biosphere, particularly the "infamous" ozone. In fact, it has been shown that VOCs are involved in the formation (or reduction) of ozone levels in the lower layers of the earth's atmosphere. Among the VOCs, monoterpenes account for about 15 percent of all organic compounds produced by plants on the planet, while isoprene can reach up to 50 percent. In the presence of pollutants typically produced in urban or industrial areas—like nitrogen oxides resulting from the massive use of fossil fuels—VOCs undergo oxidation and simultaneously catalyze the formation of ozone, which, of course, is not desirable: ozone should stay in its place, in the ozone layer (9 or 10 to 25 or 30 miles from the earth's surface), in order to intercept harmful radiation from the sun and the cosmos.

But in the absence of gaseous pollutants, such as in rural areas with low anthropization or in more natural areas such as parks and large forest complexes, the oxidation of VOCs leads to a reduction in ozone content in the troposphere. Therefore, more natural environments contribute to the reduction of greenhouse gases, lowering the amount of ozone present in the bottom layers of the atmosphere.

Bioclimatologists have gone on to try to identify the plant species that emit the largest quantities of monoterpenes and/or isoprene, so as to better assess the extent to which plants are able to reduce or, in polluted urban areas, increase the greenhouse effect in a specific geographical context. Their interest has been directed especially toward tree species, because they have a greater productive biomass. From these studies, we were able to draw some conclusions on the botanical species (and thus also on forest formations) of the most interest for the practice of forest bathing, because they release monoterpenes in significant amounts. Often these species are quite common in many natural environments, as well as in parks or urban green space in big and small cities.

Here we propose a brief review of tree species that, while not entirely exhaustive, can provide useful information for those interested in forest bathing. Moreover, remember that studies on the potential emissivity of monoterpenes by plants are now being conducted all over the world and are frequently updated with new data and information. One of the most studied areas is that of the Mediterranean basin. Among the species to be considered for their high release potential, we would mention in particular the holm oak (*Quercus ilex*), cork oak (*Quercus suber*), and kermes oak (*Quercus coccifera*). Another very important forest species is the beech (*Fagus sylvatica*), especially for its widespread distribution across the European continent, from the Scandinavian countries to southern Italy, from Normandy to Ukraine. In addition, beech forests are often forest formations of great beauty and environmental value: it is no coincidence that UNESCO has recently added the oldest beech forests of the Apennine Mountains, in Italy, to its World Heritage sites. With a somewhat less emissive potential, yet still interesting for their presence and diffusion in many natural and seminatural European environments, the following species should also be mentioned:

- chestnut (*Castanea sativa*)
- black alder (*Alnus glutinosa*)
- umbrella pine (*Pinus pinea*)
- Aleppo pine (*Pinus halepensis*)

- Scots pine (*Pinus sylvestris*)
- Norway spruce (*Picea abies*)
- silver birch (*Betula pendula*)
- European larch (*Larix decidua*)
- aspen (*Populus tremula*)
- eucalyptus (*Eucalyptus globulus*)

The European silver fir (*Abies alba*) also holds some interest, not so much because it is a high-emissive species as for the fact that it is one of the trees with greater leaf biomass, therefore able to "manufacture" a not-unremarkable amount of monoterpenes through its own photosynthetic activity. In North America, the number of forest species to be considered is as large as in Europe. Many are conifers: the Florida pine or slash pine (*Pinus elliotti*), widespread in the southeastern United States, partially overlapping with the loblolly pine (*Pinus taeda*); the spruce (*Picea abies*), native to Europe but widely introduced and naturalized in the northeast, and from the Pacific coast to the Rocky Mountains, as well as in southeastern Canada; the majestic Douglas fir (*Pseudotsuga menziesii*), native to the northwestern United States and southwestern Canada, which compensates for a middling monoterpene emission capacity with a huge leaf biomass; in the mountain areas to the east and north of the Douglas fir, the Engelmann fir (*Picea engelmannii*) is a widespread high-emissive species.

We could mention many other species of conifers, from *Abies balsamea* to *Pinus ponderosa*, *Pinus strobus*, and *Pinus sylvestris*, but we want to give enough prominence to certain equally interesting deciduous trees from this geographical area. You might encounter the red maple (*Acer rubrum*), commonly found especially in the eastern United States, from the Great Lakes region to Florida, or the hazel pine or sweetgum (*Liquidambar straciflua*), originating in the southeastern United States, though not well suited for a barefoot walk in the woods, given the "unfriendly" shape and texture of its fruit.

For their diffusion at the geographical level, two other North American deciduous trees, *Acer saccharinum* and *Populus tremuloides*, should also be mentioned, although both have a lower emission potential. The list can extend further, to include the flora of other continents: how could we leave out the numerous species of eucalyptus in the Australian forests, whose production of monoterpenes (mainly eucalyptol) is the reason for the color taken on by the atmosphere over the treetops of the aptly named Blue Mountains in New South Wales. In fact, our planet has many more "blue mountains" than you might imagine: for example, the Great Smoky Mountains and the Blue Ridge Mountains in the Appalachians owe their names to the same diffused light effect caused by the thick aerosol of these substances. These are true forest bathing paradises.

Data on the potential of the different species is mostly expressed as an emission rate, that is, the quantity of monoterpenes released by the leaves within a given interval of time. To be more precise, this rate is typically expressed in micrograms of monoterpenes per gram of dry leaf matter in one hour. This parameter shows us that, given the same environmental conditions, the more leaf mass a tree has, the higher the amount of monoterpenes it can release at a given moment. A small tree, no matter how high its specific emission rate may be, has a modest leaf mass, so we cannot expect it to produce a large amount of aromas in comparison to its surface unit.

Meanwhile, the Japanese conifer *Cryptomeria japonica* is a species that has a very low emission rate, considerably lower than those of the species listed above, but under normal development conditions it is a tree that can reach 130 feet of height, so its leaf biomass is huge, up to more than 2 kilograms per square meter of forest. For this reason, low-emissive *Cryptomeria* is able to release a quantity of monoterpenes in a surface and time unit comparable to that of the highest-emissive tree species. We could make similar considerations for other species that don't have a particularly high emission rate but a substantial leaf mass per unit area, such as the conifer *Pseudotsuga menziesii* or the *Sequoia sempervirens*.

Furthermore, the environmental conditions that influence the emission rhythms of VOCs must be taken into account. In the first part of this chapter we saw that there are plants that do not possess anatomical structures for accumulating essential oils. They are thus released into the air as the plant produces them, with an emission that is strongly dependent on the temperature of the air and the amount of light. The beech (*Fagus sylvatica*), for example, is a plant with no storage facilities, like many other deciduous trees in the Northern Hemisphere. This species grows in Europe in primarily mountainous environments, often in exposure conditions that see it prevail on the chilliest slopes. A beautiful beech forest, with adult trees and sufficiently expansive foliage, suggests a high production of monoterpenes. But if the forest formation is located on a slope that is completely exposed to the north (or to the south in the Southern Hemisphere), therefore generally colder and with a low amount of sun exposure during most of the day, it is likely that its emission of volatile substances will be less substantial than might be expected. Numerous bioclimatic studies support these claims.

The degree of development of the forest's population, the size and shape of the trees, the density and height of the foliage, the type of exposure and temperature trends are all factors to be taken into consideration to estimate actual emissive potential. For species with anatomical accumulation structures (resin ducts, glandular hairs, and so on), air temperature is more important, while exposure to optimal lighting conditions is less important. For an extensive search of suitable forest bathing environments, because of these different factors, it would be necessary to rely on an expert who can estimate a forest's potential emissivity with sufficient reliability. But don't worry—it's still possible to reap the benefits of forest bathing with the general knowledge you've gleaned here. If an advanced forest formation has at least one of the species listed above, with adult trees provided with a wide crown and healthy foliage that is evenly distributed and well exposed to the sun for a good part of the day, we can already plan a nice "forest bath" with some confidence.

We also want to keep in mind the fundamental importance of accessibility. The inclusion of trails or paths that allow you to spend at least two or three hours in the woods without getting bored or lost, structured in such a way as to allow a walk or a hike in safety without particular physical training, is certainly an important factor to consider.

Many large forests in temperate areas, nature reserves, and other protected wildlife areas, as well as peri-urban forests where tree species producing monoterpenes are prevalent, may constitute the ideal "gym" for this practice. Often these are areas where there is already a network of trails built for hiking purposes. However, there are not many natural or semi-natural areas where a system of pedestrian paths designed for forest bathing has been specially designed and organized. One of the first ever applications was created in 2015 in Italy: the Zegna Oasis, a natural pre-alpine area located in Piedmont. Given the importance of natural landscapes, it's our hope that we'll begin to see more curated areas like it.

FOREST BATHING AT THE ZEGNA OASIS

In this huge protected park created in the 1930s by the textile entrepreneur Ermenegildo Zegna, we personally conducted in 2014 a series of evaluations on the vegetation. We examined the existing tree species (beech in particular), the density of their foliage, how much sunlight they need, the prevailing winds, and other variables that could influence the outcome of walks through the woods, including ease of access and duration. In choosing the routes, we also considered the psychoemotional contribution of the environment, offering the excursionist a certain variety in the typology of the landscapes to cross. The result was a detailed study for estimating the trees' emission potential. It allowed us to identify three circular paths ideal for forest bathing, where readers would be able to take in the highest concentration of positive monoterpenes. Adequate signage informs and accompanies the visitor along all the paths. Moreover, you can combine this visit with the bioenergetic experience of the Bosco del Sorriso (described in chapter 7, "The Bioenergetic Landscape").

6. NEGATIVE IONS AND NATURAL ENVIRONMENTS

Human evolution took place inside the ecosphere, that part of the biosphere where environmental conditions allow for the formation and development of ecosystems. In relation to the earth's radius, which is 3,959 miles, the biosphere is so thin one can think of it as a sort of covering film for our planet. Over the last two hundred years, humans have poured all the waste produced by their enormous technological progress into it. The level of pollution we have reached can be conveyed with a single figure: in 2015, for the first time in *Homo sapiens*' history, carbon dioxide, the most well known of the greenhouse gases, passed the threshold of 400 parts per million in the air.

Among the chemophysical properties of the biosphere that humanity has altered in recent times, the air's level of ionization is not debated enough. Human intervention has affected this specific environmental parameter in various ways, creating—especially in urban spaces—atmospheric conditions that differ greatly from those in which humankind has historically evolved.

Today we live in domestic and work environments where the quality and quantity of ions present in the air we breathe (and in which we carry out the vast majority of our activities) is very poor. This scarcity is not without its health effects, according to the results of numerous scientific studies.

Ionization of the Air as an Index of Environmental Quality

The expression "ionization" refers to the quantity and the quality of electrically charged particles in the atmosphere. Even hundreds of years ago, there were some who theorized the existence of a force in the air that had an effect on animals and human beings. The first true experiments on atmospheric electricity date back to Benjamin Franklin in the 1700s. Around the same time, Italian mathematician and physicist Giovanbattista Beccaria formulated the first theory that "nature makes ample use of atmospheric electricity."

It was not until the end of the twentieth century, however, that the existence of ions in the air was proven. The first groundbreaking experiments were conducted in Germany by Julius Elster and Hans Geitel and in the United Kingdom by Joseph John Thomson; but it was the University of California, Berkeley, biometeorologist Albert P. Krueger who began studying the biological properties of negative ions in the 1970s. The earth's atmosphere is a decidedly complex medium, endowed with forces that interact with the planet's surface to create electrical environments that vary across space and time. Thus the widespread presence of electrical charges in the biosphere is perfectly natural.

At ground level, a significant portion of ions is generated by natural radioactivity, such as the decay of radium (a radioactive element contained in the earth's crust) into radon gas. Above the oceans and tall mountains, cosmic radiation and the sun's ultraviolet irradiation also act as major ionizing agents. These phenomena are joined by many others distributed unevenly over the planet's surface, such as storms, thunder, friction generated by the movement of large air masses, atmospheric turbulence, volcanic eruptions, waterfalls and large bodies of water that flow or crash against solid surfaces, the presence of pointed objects that accumulate electric charges, chemical reactions produced in plant tissue by photosynthesis, and so on.

A common characteristic among these phenomena is having a certain amount of energy that causes molecules in the mixture of gases in the air to release an electron, which is immediately attracted to another molecule, giving it a negative charge and forming a negative ion (also called an "anion"), while the original molecule becomes, in turn, a positive ion. Some particles of water vapor and other free atoms of atmospheric gas quickly group around these primary ions to form so-called "small ions" in the air.

Solid and liquid particles in suspension or transported by wind, such as some pollutants, can also become electrically charged. However, these are called "secondary atmospheric ions" or "intermediate and large ions" because of their greater dimensions.

When size exceeds ten thousandths of a millimeter (0.1 micrometers) we are no longer dealing with ions but with electrically charged aerosols. Small ions, having a diameter at least a thousand times smaller, are for this reason more mobile and biologically active, while large ions are much less mobile and generally inactive or even harmful from a biological perspective. The earth's surface is predominately endowed with a negative charge, which tends to repel the air's small negative ions, which rapidly move away from the ground (the opposite, of course, happens with small positive ions). This occurs in sufficiently open spaces and in the absence of significant tree cover over the ground. In contrast, it has been observed that in natural environments characterized by well-developed plant life, in particular trees and shrubs, negative ions predominate over the positive. Not only that, the total quantity of ions in the air is also greater in a large complex of flora compared with air in areas transformed by humans or other areas with little to no vegetation.

Let us clarify that small ions have an extremely short lifespan, from a fraction of one second to a just a few seconds, after which they recombine with ions that have an opposite charge. They may also be absorbed by intermediate or large ions (which are more stable), or lose their charge by coming into contact with a solid or liquid surface. However, their production continues as long as the energy conditions to activate the process persist; thus, the average ion content in the air of a specific environment is a result of this dynamic equilibrium.

When the air in a certain place is affected by solid or liquid particles coming from human activity, such as residential heating, industrial processes, and motor vehicle emissions, "nuclei" of condensation are formed, which attract smaller ions and produce electrically charged (positive or negative) aerosol particles.

This liquid-gas mixture tends to hover in the lower layers of the atmosphere, precisely where people are most present. The polluted particles and water vapor molecules stratify to the point of turning the air a sickly yellow, with a great reduction in horizontal visibility, forming smog. Highly polluted urban or industrial spaces are thus extremely poor in small ions.

In indoor environments it is primarily electric and electronic machinery that capture ions, especially those with a negative charge. Even the presence of smoke contributes to reducing the number of small ions in the air. A major reduction is also caused by air-conditioning systems, with the absorption of charged particles in the filters and motors. Finally, in car interiors, where air is confined and electric and electronic equipment are surrounded by surfaces made with synthetic materials, you can see a very high reduction in small ions and a simultaneous spread of dust particles, which are not exactly healthy for our lungs. In general, the depletion of negative ions in urban environments is greater than that of positive ions, because they are more easily pushed away or removed from the air.

To get a better idea, let's look at the average ion content in the air of various types of environments, natural and manmade. The data illustrated here has been gathered from several sources, so it refers not only to different environments but also to survey and measurement conditions that often differ from one another. Rather than absolute values, which can vary greatly across space and time, it is helpful to observe the respective proportions of the ionic contents.

TYPE OF ENVIRONMENT	NEGATIVE IONS PER CM³	POSITIVE IONS PER CM³	TOTAL IONS PER CM³
Environments sheltered by waterfalls	9,000–18,000	1,000–2,000	10,000–20,000
Temperate forest	1,000–2,500	800–2,000	1,800–4,500
Mountains, with pure dry air	1,500–2,000	2,000–2,500	3,500–4,500
Rural environments, open space, in fair weather conditions	500–1,500	700–1,800	1,200–3,300
Open space, before a storm	750	2,500	3,250
Open space, at the end of a storm	2,500	750	3,250
Typical office environment (indoors)	50–150	100–200	150–350
Interior of an operating vehicle (confined space)	20–50	80–150	100–200

We should note that an atmosphere of open natural spaces (rural areas, meadows, pastures with little tree coverage, etc.) with a total absence of pollution may have between 1,500 and 4,000 ions per cubic centimeter, with a slight predominance (12 to 20 percent greater) of positive ions.

In typical forest areas in our latitudes the volume may be similar, but the relationship is reversed in favor of negative ions. In large rainforests the total ionic content in the atmosphere can be considerably higher, but the predominance of negative ions over positive remains the same.

For hundreds of thousands of years, human evolution took place primarily in these environments with similar levels of air ionization. Negative ions in particular were always abundant and readily available. Unfortunately, however, urban and indoor environments do not even come close to the ionization levels typical of more natural surroundings. We need to ask ourselves what the consequences may be for our health when we find ourselves living in places so poor in atmospheric ions, especially negative ions.

Biological Effects of Atmospheric Ions

Are negative ions really so important for our health? The scientific literature on the topic leaves no room for doubt.

Dozens of studies completed from 1975 to today from all over the world have not only demonstrated the beneficial effects of negative ionization in the air, such as cleaning the atmosphere, but also thoroughly investigated its effects on psychophysical well-being.

Asthma was one of the first diseases to be the subject of clinical experimentation in environments rich in negative ions. A few dozen minutes of exposure each day to intense negative ionization was enough to improve the entire array of patients' symptoms. In the 1980s and '90s, researchers had already reported a reduction in asthmatic conditions with a significant reduction in the administration and dosage of medications such as theophylline and cortisone.

Other studies focused on elements connected to stress, mood disorders, and physical and mental fatigue. A predominance of positive ions in the air brought with it an increase in these disturbances, while a prevalence of negative ions diminished them.

The agitation or even discomfort felt by some meteoropathic people before a storm or when certain winds are blowing (such as the Föhn in Alpine regions, the Sirocco in parts of Italy, the Santa Anas in the United States, or the Khamsin in the Middle East) is a result of the greater quantity of positive ions generated in the lower layers of the atmosphere. The aforementioned winds are shown to be disagreeable even to animals, and not only domesticated ones—if dogs and cats behave worse than their owners during these times, they are probably not doing it out of empathy with human beings but because of the increased concentration of positive ions.

The phenomenon has been extensively examined in several nations, and not only because of increased absences from work due to various symptoms such as respiratory stress, migraines, fatigue, and various other maladies. Indeed, the agitated and irritable states clearly caused by these environmental conditions have led some judges to extend greater leniency in sentences for crimes of passion. In some hospitals, elective surgery is even postponed or ionizers are employed in the operating rooms. Even some well-informed teachers know to expect less-brilliant results from their pupils during these days. In addition to consulting her horoscope, a university student, thinking about exams, might also want to check the weather forecast!

On the other hand, environments with a predominance of negative ions are shown to be effective in reducing states of stress, depression, and psychophysical maladies connected to stressful events.

Various studies and experiments have noted the antidepressant effects of high concentrations of anions in the air. A review published in the United States in 2013 presents a meta-analysis of five different clinical studies that all confirmed a direct correlation between high negative ionization of environments and improvement in depressive states. Studies conducted in Japan and Romania showed that a high concentration of negative ions in the environment (greater than 10,000 ions per cubic centimeter) enables quicker recovery from intense physical exertion, with a normalization of blood pressure in less time (moreover, evidence of the latter phenomenon for subjects with hypertension has also been shown in a number of other studies). Studies also show that cognitive performance, especially memory, is improved in both children and adults.

Even sleep disturbances can be significantly reduced when the environment is enriched with negative ions, while an excess in positive ions, as well as a scarcity in the total amount of ions in the air, produces the opposite effect. In individuals who suffer from chronic stress, positive ionization of the air does nothing but accentuate their symptoms, as well as weaken their immune defenses.

Various studies have ascertained that when positive ions in the air are absorbed by the human body, the majority transform into free radicals that can give rise to oxidation processes, increasing acidity in the body and accelerating aging and cellular degeneration. For this reason, some Japanese researchers launched lab experiments to discover to what extent treatment with anions can reduce the risk of developing cancer. Even taking into account the need for further investigations and in-depth studies, the preliminary results appear very favorable.

Protecting ourselves from the excess of positive ions in the environment is thus very important, but it is not always easy given that 80 to 85 percent of ionic particles enter the body through the skin and the remaining 15 to 20 percent through respiration. Balancing both the excess positive ionization and the low level of ionization in our environments, the best solution is still improving air quality by increasing small anions, namely, those that are most biologically active. But it would also be wise to change our lifestyles, with more time spent in natural environments, which show greater potential negative ionization.

Moreover, there is no toxicity threshold regarding the absorption of negative ions: even with anionic concentrations greater than 100,000 units per cubic centimeter, no organ malfunctions or symptoms of illness were recorded for subjects participating in clinical experiments.

Now, if negative ions are scarce in the environments where we pass most of our time, is it possible to take care of this in some way and "produce" them?

Air ionizers have been recommended (especially by their manufacturers) for purifying domestic and work environments of foul odors and pollutants. The idea that negative ions produced by a home appliance can reduce unpleasant odors in a closed space is not quite correct: doing this "dirty job" of ionization also generates a byproduct: ozone. Indeed, many devices labeled as ionizers or air purifiers have this "small" problem—that together with negative ions they emit ozone, which is widely known to be a greenhouse gas and which, more important, is an irritant for the respiratory system. Producing it at home is obviously not ideal, especially if we have small children living with us. Ozone has a characteristic strong odor, while ions have neither odor nor flavor. After all, these come from the ionization of certain molecules in the air, which is by definition an odorless, tasteless mix of gases.

Fortunately, our nose has a fairly low threshold for detecting ozone, ranging from 0.005 to 0.02 parts per million in the air, while irritation of the mucous membranes of the nose, eyes, and throat, together with headache and labored breath, arise at a concentration at least 5 to 10 times greater than this.

Not all ionizers produce ozone; some models are built so as to minimize its production. When purchasing an environmental ionizer it is a good idea to make sure the manufacturer states the level of ozone emissions: look carefully, as many companies do not.

One more tip: a good ionization device should not have air filters, because it is likely most of the ions will be absorbed by these filters, and you'll be left with a simple dust filter. In the absence of an ionizer, one can always resort to natural ventilation, opening the windows and letting the air circulate for a few minutes, especially after a storm or intense rain when the atmosphere is rich in negative ions.

The presence of plants inside our living spaces or closed

workplaces can contribute significantly to improving air quality, including ionization and reduction of pollutants. But we'll get to that later on.

In calm, sunny weather conditions, if we cannot take a walk through a park rich in tall trees or a forest area, we can at least allow ourselves a long, lovely shower each day, taking advantage in small part of what physicists call the Lenard effect (ionization due to the collision of water particles). It's not much, but it's better than passing long periods of time in an ion-poor environment without attempting to mitigate its effects.

So which natural environments are able to furnish our body with the supply of ions it needs?

A Natural Ion Shower

Wherever there are bodies of moving water there is always negative ionization, created by the Lenard or "waterfall" effect: the greater the kinetic energy with which a body of water crashes into a solid object or disperses into the air, the more notable and effective the production of ions.

The separation of electrons from water molecules, which are electrically neutral, produces as many positive ions as negative, as we have seen at the beginning of this chapter.

But while the majority of negative ions remain suspended in the air until their neutralization, positively charged water particles rapidly fall to the ground (or the body of water) after impact, and are in turn absorbed and deactivated. For this reason, the atmosphere near bodies of colliding water can contain as many as tens of thousands of small negative ions per cubic centimeter, these ions being much more active from a biological perspective as well.

The spectacular waterfalls formed by rivers large and small are an important source of negative ionization, with a high therapeutic quality. The shore of the sea or ocean can likewise be an effective source, with its power correlated to the water's degree of agitation: it is clear that a wave colliding forcefully against a cliff can produce more negative ions than a placid lake lapping a sandy shore.

Of course you don't have to take a cruise to Niagara Falls or watch the waves crash at Thunder Hole in New England's Acadia National Park to get an effective ion shower. If well planned, even small waterfalls or fountains with a flow of water comparable to a stream can fill the air in their immediate vicinity with several thousand negative ions per cubic centimeter. The important thing is that the water's movement is sufficiently high and forceful to produce a significant Lenard effect.

The body of water's beneficial activities can be further strengthened by lush greenery, with trees and shrubbery capable of holding the aerosols in the area benefiting from negative ionization. Even decorative elements such as fountains that reproduce the effect of small waterfalls can help in creating effective green spaces aimed at psychophysiological well-being.

For several years the study of air ionization has also been extended to hydrothermal areas. Hot springs have biological and therapeutic properties due especially to their chemical composition and in part to their temperature. A thermal or hyperthermal complex in which waters circulate and bubble so as to release a high amount of aerosols into the air is definitely a significant source of small anions.

If you aren't near an active body of water, other sources of negative ions accessible to anyone are natural environments characterized by sufficiently dense, lush vegetation and a prevalent, well-developed tree cover. The ideal model would be a rainforest with the lower density of a temperate forest. It isn't difficult to find this model: many deciduous and coniferous forests can have these characteristics, as long as there is enough water to guarantee good levels of relative humidity in the air. A good amount of natural light is favorable, thanks to the generation of negative ions during photosynthesis.

We can also infer that many forest environments suitable for the practice of forest bathing also have a sufficient level of air ionization, often with a predominance of negative ions over positive ones.

If the forests are located in a mountain environment, it is likely that the amount of small anions is even more significant. There is also a natural tendency for negative ions to distance themselves from the earth's surface, so those produced in adjacent foothill areas also "transit" through these higher altitudes.

Furthermore, there is another phenomenon found more frequently in mountainous areas that leads to air ionization. This is the "corona effect," characterized by objects with a pointed shape such as certain mountain peaks or especially sharp rocks. Background radiation can bring greater potential energy to the point of an object exposed to open air, creating a spontaneous release of electrons.

These negatively charged atmospheric nitrogen and oxygen molecules initiate a chain reaction that lasts as long as the potential energy present at the pointed tip remains high.

These different elements explain why a greater concentration of ions is recorded high in the mountains as opposed to, for example, an area with open fields.

Waterfalls, seashores, large bodies of moving water, hot springs, forests, woods, mountains: nature gives us a wide array of therapeutic opportunities.

The forest bath and ion shower are two examples of the purifying, regenerative power of natural environments. Now it's time to explore a new resource provided exclusively by contact with plant energy.

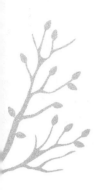

The first thing that comes to mind when we think of nature is probably a tree. It's an important and often majestic presence that evokes a sense of tranquillity and well-being. However, we still know very little about what actually happens at a biological level when we touch a tree. Are there physical reactions within the human body? What happens to the tree? Could plants have an influence on our habitat's quality of life?

Thanks to a body of research that has allowed us to obtain results that previously would have been impossible, we can provide a concrete, increasingly precise answer to these questions and others, offering perspectives that could alter our very relationship with nature. All of this is made possible by applying a new way of studying the relationship between plants and humans from an *energetic* point of view.

Hugging Trees: Just a New Age Thing?

In many ancient cultures, trees were a highly significant symbol. Thanks to their astonishing vitality and longevity, trees and other plants have often been considered objects of worship and respect, home to divinities, grantors of favors and health, and thus "sacred." Even thaumaturgical powers have been attributed to certain specimens, reinforcing the archetypal image of the "healing" tree that can directly influence human well-being.

Traces of these convictions can be found in all ancient traditions, including Vedic, Chinese, Aboriginal, and Native American, and in groups of people who have preserved deep connections with nature, such as Amazonian tribes. In these cultures, the tradition of physical contact with trees is still alive. It is a ritualistic and symbolic gesture, but also therapeutic, practiced with the aim of generating a real exchange of energy, replenishing vital force, and strengthening character. Just over a century ago, European medical culture still held the idea that being in contact with a sizable tree could help the body and the mind, and similar traditions have been passed on until recently in the rural cultures of many parts of the world.

Today many of these ancient teachings have been reclaimed, with varying degrees of awareness, within numerous cultural movements that are alternative or simply conscious of a deeper dialogue with nature.

"Tree hugging" is an increasingly widespread practice that leaves a tangible sense of psychophysical well-being in those who practice it. Yet contemporary society, particularly the scientific community, is largely unprepared for such unconventional behavior and its implications. The majority of people are still indifferent to it, if not skeptical or derisive. Perhaps there have been times that you have felt the desire to touch or hug a tree, compelled by an instinctive, empathetic pull, but you probably felt embarrassed. However, the emotional aspect alone does not explain the sense of well-being resulting from such contact. What is behind this deep-rooted connection?

For some time now, this topic has fascinated researchers around the world, who have attempted a scientific explanation for the intuitions of so many nature lovers. The prestigious HeartMath Institute (HMI) in California has proposed, with a project called Interconnectivity Tree Research Project, to extend existing research on the topic by looking into possible forms of interaction with plants and studying the effects that this interaction has on people. It is increasingly evident that the beneficial consequences of contact with trees and plants do not only concern the mind but also involve the energetic properties of humans. Researchers, however, have encountered difficulties when trying to understand the actual dynamics of this relationship and how to measure it adequately.

In order to deepen our knowledge on the subject, then, we need to consider electromagnetism, a form of energy that supports all living processes and allows both humans and plants to relate instantly with the world around us within the biosphere.

Biosphere, Energy, and Electromagnetism

Let's imagine a vast and complex laboratory in which millions of chemical, physical, electromagnetic, nuclear, and gravitational processes are happening constantly. This is the biosphere: an extremely thin shell that surrounds our planet, which hosts all forms of life that populate planet Earth, from the depths of the oceans up to 32,000 feet in the air. An environment in dynamic balance, a large organism—as James Lovelock interpreted it in his Gaia hypothesis—that has allowed life to manifest and evolve, maintaining the ideal characteristics for living and carrying out vital processes for millions of years. However, this does not change the fact that there are notable differences in quality between the places in which we live. These variations are in part linked to natural phenomena, such as the climate or ionization, and in part to increasingly invasive human behaviors.

In this large shell, which is diverse and variable, human beings need not only ideal environmental conditions but also an adequate source of vital energy, the invisible nourishment that makes the difference between a living body and a dead one. "Without energy, life would switch off immediately and cell tissues would collapse," the Nobel laureate Albert Szent-Györgyi confirmed. But where does this vital energy come from, and what feeds it?

Everybody knows that humans can survive for a while without food and water, but we cannot live a single moment without the energy supply of the sun. We receive electromagnetic radiation in various wavelengths from the sun, particularly light and infrared, which nourish and enable life on Earth, warming us and enabling plants to produce oxygen and organic material through photosynthesis. The sun also creates a powerful magnetic field, which in turn conditions the geomagnetic field of the Earth and its fluctuations. Then factor in the effects of the gravitation of celestial bodies and the enormous rotation of our galaxy.

Like the inside of a giant watch, the energies of the cosmos create rhythms and pulsations in living and nonliving materials. In the third century BC Greek botanist Theophrastus suggested cutting wood at the start of the waning moon in order to obtain a more durable material. The effectiveness of this practice has recently been proven by a study carried out at the University of Zurich.

In the 1950s Giorgio Piccardi observed, through thousands of experiments repeated around the world, that the energetic influence of the sun and the cycle of seasons changed chemical reactions and the precipitation of compounds. This compelled other researchers to verify similar fluctuations in human and botanical behavior.

These phenomena are made possible by various manifestations of electromagnetic forces that are at the base of the structure of matter. We could also think of them as the fundamental biological language that nature uses to allow each element, from the atoms that make up the material to the more complex structures of living beings, to interact and instantaneously transmit the information that regulates vital processes.

Everything vibrates, and does so with specific characteristics and objectives. In a now famous quote, Nikola Tesla stated, "If you want to understand the secrets of the universe, think in terms of energy, frequency and vibration."

Immersed in this pulsating ocean, living beings have developed remarkable sensitivities to electromagnetic waves. It is a phenomenon that is evident in many animal species: sharks, rays, and catfish, for example, are able to sense and respond to extremely weak intensities of electric fields in order to find food over long distances. As for humans, pronounced physical reactions have been observed in some hypersensitive people when they are exposed to very weak intensities of certain electromagnetic frequencies. Biological sensitivity applies to all living beings to varying extents. It's as if we are able to tune in to an almost imperceptible radio signal, while avoiding the interferences of nearby stations. This selectivity is a good thing, because to be sensitive to all the fields of energy in which we are immersed would be rather overwhelming.

In this way, the cells of human beings are comparable to small celestial bodies: they give off and receive a large quantity of signals such as radio waves, microwaves, and visible and invisible light waves, as well as infrasound, which all communicate necessary vital information. Carlo Ventura, a biology professor at the University of Bologna who conducts innovative research on stem cells, explains: "We have become aware that cells are capable of emitting electromagnetic fields and nanomechanical vibrations. This has led us to discover that exposure to radio electric fields can 'reprogram' even non-stem adult human cells, such as dermal fibroblasts, into types of cells they would not otherwise transform into, such as cardiovascular, neuronal, and muscular cells. These results show that the destiny of stem cells can be noticeably altered by physical energy."

All of the above means that, in our environment, life is closely connected to electromagnetism, and this phenomenon can act directly—and selectively—on how humans, animals, and plants function.

The Living Organism as Biological Antenna

In 1960, Walter Kunnen founded Archibo Biologica in Antwerp, Belgium, the first research center to specialize in the influences of the biosphere on living things and the study of bioenergetics. Kunnen was a tenacious scholar who thought outside the box. This was, perhaps, how he succeeded in developing a decisively original research method that was surprisingly precise in evaluating the quality of the environment and measuring the effects that it produces on the various functions of living organisms.

He started off by thoroughly investigating the practical applications of bioresonance, a field based on the theory that every substance oscillates principally on its own specific frequency. In the 1950s, this discipline saw its first practical applications in the field of medicine. Kunnen's interest in biology led him to demonstrate that every group or collection of cells with the same function, liver cells for example, resonates on precise electromagnetic frequencies, allowing the organs to gather the energy they need to survive. This principle is identical to that of an antenna that receives or sends a certain electromagnetic signal. When this "antenna function" is interrupted, the body ceases to live. In living beings, we can also observe examples of organs or systems with an antenna function: in animals the eye carries out this magnificent task, converting light radiation into electrical stimuli for the brain, and in green leaves chloroplasts absorb light and activate the process of photosynthesis.

Kunnen wanted to understand the effects on living beings of being constantly immersed in a biosphere full of electromagnetic signals on all frequencies, and how to distinguish the useful and harmful information these signals offer us. This was a feasible operation, but it depended on a new comprehension of energy phenomena in biology, as well as an adequate measuring instrument.

Cellular Nutrition and Health

Electromagnetism is a phenomenon well studied by physicists, but even today science finds its limits in the biological interpretation of phenomena like electricity, magnetism, and gravity, even if their mechanical effects can be measured and predicted. For example, it is still difficult to establish precisely which effects are produced in our bodies when we are exposed to one of the many sources of electrosmog, such as cell phone towers or high-voltage power lines. In light of this, Kunnen proposed a different vision of electromagnetism, certainly outside the conventional box, but very functional in terms of biology. This understanding will help us understand the mechanisms through which we can study our interaction with plants.

According to Kunnen's experiment, what is usually called

an electromagnetic wave is actually made up of a pair of spirals that move forward in space intertwined together. One rotates to the right (clockwise rotation with positive polarity) and the other to the left (counterclockwise rotation with negative polarity). These fields transport information within the biosphere and at the same time give energy to living beings as carrier waves and carried waves. The carrier waves emitted by a radio station, for example, are the radio signal that transports in space the various transmissions (the information, or carried waves) that we receive when we listen. In the same way, in nature there are carrying and carried waves that, as we will see later on, are of fundamental biological importance.

Carrier waves are signals that move through space in a straight line, have neutral or balanced polarity (because the positive and negative spirals they are composed of are of the same intensity), and act as vectors or "modes of transport" in space for carried waves, which are electromagnetic fields with frequencies that resonate and interact with the various organs of the human body. These are often "unbalanced," because their spirals of positive and negative polarity are of different intensities, which are conditioned by many factors. And it is this characteristic that determines the diverse information— beneficial or harmful—sent to cells. But why is polarity so important in biology?

To explain, Kunnen proposed an energetic representation of the cell, which can help us understand how it is nourished both in terms of chemistry and electromagnetism. His measurements showed him that the healthy cell, if examined in its own natural environment, is a dynamic structure that tends to maintain a predominantly negative charge on the surface of the membrane, while the inside (called cellular light) is predominantly positive, unlike what is assumed in biology. Since we know that opposite magnetic poles attract and like poles repel, according to this model the healthy cell is nourished by principally attracting useful substances that promote a positive polarity. The cell does not live in a static magnetic field, but emits its own specific frequency and other electromagnetic signals that enter into resonance with nourishing elements. This allows it to dynamically attract and modulate its nutrition through a phenomenon that we could therefore call electromagnetic osmosis.

For the same reason, if a cell is hit by an electromagnetic field with which it enters into resonance (carried wave) and which has a greater intensity on its negative polarity, the cellular membrane inverts its own external charge through magnetic repulsion and loses its polarity, which damages the cell.

Exposure to fields that have greater intensities on positive polarity tend to play a rebalancing or even therapeutic role, reinforcing the correct functionality and health of the cell, since opposite poles attract.

Kunnen's cellular energetic model plays a fundamental role in our understanding of the biological significance of electromagnetism and its implications for daily life. But his investigations of the biosphere and subtle electromagnetic mechanisms wouldn't have been possible without a simple instrument invented in the 1950s.

The Lecher Antenna

The Lecher antenna, named in homage to the Austrian engineer Ernst Lecher and invented by German physicist Reinhard Schneider, was designed to accurately measure electromagnetic wavelengths and frequencies of biological interest, without adding any energies or distorting the measured signal.

This instrument allows the user to select a desired frequency to receive a signal (just like on a regular radio) whose sensitivity is part of the microwave field. By following a precise measurement technique, it is possible to amplify the vibration or electromagnetic resonance of the antenna to the sensitive biological structure of the human organism. The antenna used by Kunnen and his collaborators is an enhanced version of Schneider's, and allows the user to take highly detailed measurements of the intensity of the electromagnetic fields at each of its two polarities. This is extremely important, because it is the variable that defines the biological quality of the signals the cell encounters. Practical experiments have indeed demonstrated that cellular health requires a well-defined and even relationship between these intensities, with a slight predominance of the dextrorotatory component (positive polarity). On the other hand we could have aggressive signals, or signals too weak to carry energetic nourishment, or therapeutic signals, as in the case of a strong dextrorotatory predominance.

The Lecher antenna, if used correctly, is still the most simple, versatile, and sophisticated biological measuring system. Its practicality lies in the fact that it does not need software or an electronic circuit to function, but only the correct and precise training of the operator to react to the electromagnetic microimpulses provoked by contact with the antenna. This equipment allows us to carry out analysis on the energetic state of various human organs in a short time. It also allows us to measure its reactions to environmental influences and verify the existence of electromagnetic fields in nature that are extremely weak but of extremely high biological affinity.

Bioenergetic Landscape: The Bioenergetic Study of Trees

Walter Kunnen's discoveries and his original investigative method with the Lecher antenna made it possible to embark on a research project that brings humans closer to plants in a surprising way. The outcome of this experiment is the "bioenergetic landscape," a technique that studies and uses the energetic properties of trees to create green spaces that are particularly favorable to our well-being. But how is it possible to foster a concrete interaction between humans and plants? How close is the affinity between such different creatures?

Plants have long been used for therapeutic purposes in medicine and phytotherapy (the use of plant-based medications in the treatment of disease), but knowledge of the role that they can play in our health from an energetic viewpoint has only recently reemerged. After all, the electromagnetic mechanisms that permit animal life are the same that rule botanical life. Plants give off weak electromagnetic fields just as humans do. Now, seeing as every electromagnetic field conveys information, even the ones produced by a tree, for example, can be measured and interpreted.

The discovery of electric currents inside plants has many illustrious precursors, from Jagadish Chandra Bose to Harold Saxton Burr and Vladimir Rajda, who have authored very interesting studies on the topic. Nevertheless, this is no surprise to biochemists or those who know anything about electrophysiology; it might even seem obvious.

The bioenergetic analysis of trees has allowed us to cross the boundary of physiology into the field of energetic biology. We can now recognize properties that have been unknown or merely imagined until now, that drive us to connect with the botanical world in a more conscious way that is extraordinarily useful for our existence.

Plants, like humans, emit biological frequencies

Apart from the evident physical differences, trees have a strong energetic resemblance to humans. In fact, each plant is an antenna that vibrates and emits electromagnetic signals at frequencies that are in resonance with our organs. This does not mean, for example, that plants have a heart or a stomach, but we can hypothesize that they possess cells or common biological systems that are organized in a way that is energetically similar to humans. We can also hypothesize that they probably carry out a similar function, or in some cases an even more "specialized" one, enabling the plant's survival, albeit in different ways. In addition to what we could define (at least energetically) as the plant nervous system, we can measure the existence of immune, circulatory, and lymphatic systems, as well as that of sexual function, and more. It is therefore possible to carry out an energetic diagnosis of plants using the Lecher antenna to obtain information about their state of health, measuring the intensity and biological quality of some of the organ frequencies that we use for humans. Recent discoveries made by the Laboratorio Internazionale di Neurobiologia Vegetale (International Laboratory for Plant Neurobiology) at the Science Center of the University of Florence directed by Stefano Mancuso have proven as much.

Professor Mancuso's study on the ability of root apexes to perceive many environmental parameters that allow them to express sensitivity, memory, and a refined form of intelligence, despite not having a brain, is also very telling. These studies, among others, support and scientifically elaborate on Charles Darwin's hypotheses on plant sensitivity and the experiments conducted by the physicist Jagadish Chandra Bose in Calcutta in the early twentieth century. The functional, if not structural, similarities between the cells that make up the animal nervous system and those of the root apex could derive from an early close connection between living beings. After all, plants were the first multicellular organisms to inhabit this planet billions of years ago, and all the subsequent complex living forms became differentiated starting with plants.

Plants possess specific energetic characteristics

The biodiversity expressed by each plant is not only structural or functional, but also biochemical and energetic, and this is highly important in terms of the interaction that it can have with our own health. Indeed, plants emit bioelectromagnetic fields that are able to influence the state of our organs to varying extents. Each type or species of tree, for example, tends to express its "energetic personality," which is manifested in the form of signals that are extremely weak but highly resonant for our organism. So there are some very beneficial plants, whose biological quality can even reach the maximum measurable value with the Lecher antenna, and others that have less favorable or even harmful effects at the bioenergetic level. For example, lindens emit very beneficial signals for all organs, but with a superior intensity on the nervous and lymphatic systems and mucous membranes. Beeches also produce generally beneficial effects, but usually have the greatest affinity with different organs, for example the prostate, ovaries, cardiovascular system, and small intestine.

Within one genus (*Quercus, Prunus, Magnolia*, etc.) we can also find a variety of energetic characteristics. For example, within the *Prunus* genus there are species that are very beneficial for the organism, such as the common cherry, peach, almond, and apricot trees. But there is also the cherry laurel (*Prunus laurocerasus*), which is not at all favorable to our organism as it emits mainly signals with a strong negative polarity.

The measurements taken thus far with the Lecher antenna have come from many genera and species of arboreal and decorative plants, allowing us to trace a general line of the bioenergetic characteristics of the most common botanical groups. For example, of the plants studied that are widespread in Europe and the United States, those considered highly beneficial are the following: Acer (maples), apple, ash, bay, beech, birch, boxwood, camellia, cedar, cherry, chestnut, dogwood, elder, elm, eucalyptus, European nettle tree, ginkgo, holly, holm oak, hornbeam, horse chestnut, juniper, linden, liquidambar, magnolia, myrtle, oak, olive, palm, pine, plane, pomegranate, redwood, rosemary, spruce, strawberry tree, and willow. Some of those, on the other hand, that are considered disruptive to some extent are: cherry laurel, crepe myrtle, cypress, oleander, walnut, yew, and to varying extents ficus, except for the common fig (fruit-bearing fig). The most common fruit plants are generally beneficial except for the walnut, as mentioned above.

Tree Energies and Health

The manifestation of a specific electromagnetic identity is a phenomenon that characterizes trees and plants more than animals or humans. Their substantially (but only apparently) static nature implies that they can maintain a more or less stable regulatory system. Therefore they have developed capacities for response and adaptation to the environment that are much more complex than those of humans. A study published in *Science* showed that the common wheat genome is made up of around 106,000 genes, the rice genome almost 50,000, and the human genome "only" 20,000. The researchers state that this is because "plants have to solve problems, while we humans can avoid them." On the other hand, movement and the consequent metabolic dynamism of animals means their energetic state is always in flux, thus dependent on many factors.

Yet even if the same types of plants maintain their beneficial properties everywhere, various elements can change the intensity and quality of their bioenergetic emissions. From one place to another the chemistry of the soil changes, as well as the nutrients absorbed, climate, quantity of light absorbed, exposure to various forms of physical and electromagnetic pollution, and interactions, positive or not, with nearby plants (allelobiosis). All these characteristics can explain, but also condition, the expression and energetic quality of each plant.

Analysis with the Lecher antenna shows us that, even if weakened, trees continue to be generous dispensers of healthy energies, as long as they're not in severe distress. All trees are able to express extreme contentment and vitality if surrounded by a healthy environment. Unfortunately this is less and less frequently the case, which humans have, in large measure, to answer for.

Hugging Trees: A Healthy Practice

Numerous measurements of different trees and people in various places on the planet have shown that hugging or even just touching a tree is not merely providing a direct link with a solid and majestic living being, nor is it just a trendy New Age suggestion, nor merely a useful practice to earth or "ground" static electricity built up in the body. Having physical contact with a tree, as with any plant, however big or small, is the simplest way to instantly provoke a bioelectromagnetic or bioenergetic reaction that is measurable in our bodies. If the tree is beneficial, we can compare the intensity and quality of this response to when we consume a drug, food, or any other substance taken as therapy. The effect is purely energetic, but is sufficient to stimulate and nourish our vital processes.

At the same time, contact with humans causes an energetic feedback loop that sends our complex biological information— that which defines us as humans—back into the tree. It is truly fascinating to measure the tree's immediate reaction to this contact.

Trees love contact with humans. Plants often react very favorably to an aware and compassionate touch. For example, the oak responds with enthusiasm to the hug with a positive effect on all our organs, especially the nervous and immune systems, ovaries, adrenal glands, and the thyroid. The most exciting thing, however, is seeing what happens when a child hugs a tree. The plant reacts with an impressive response, sending signals of great positivity (i.e., dextrorotatory) into space on the frequencies of its own immune and nervous systems. We should perhaps ask ourselves what the tree really "feels" in the absence of complex neurological structures, as well as why and with which senses all this can happen. We should not forget that humans too sometimes perceive something similar, which has a lot to do with feelings, as long as the most instinctive and authentic part of our being is allowed to emerge. Is it perhaps worth exploring "plant consciousness"? Without falling into anthropomorphism, or into an anthropocentric scientific and philosophical perspective, it may be worth exploring this peculiar and refined sensibility, so close to a sort of "vegetal conscience."

The intense reciprocity of reactions that arises from simple human-tree contact is also proof that we are in fact connected to nature in a circular way. Frequently hugging trees could therefore be considered a therapeutic and stimulating practice, a type of energetic and even emotional medicine, in which real biological impact can be measured. Could we encourage these kinds of practice in our cities, offering cultural and scientific support for them?

Absolutely, as long as we construct new educational foundations and more mindful lifestyles. It was truly a pleasure to see the sign placed some years ago at the entrance to the Royal Botanic Garden in Sydney that invited visitors to hug trees and walk barefoot on the grass.

But how close should we get to feel the effects of these energetic fields? Usually the weak intensity of electromagnetic fields emitted by trees produces significantly measurable effects on the human body at up to 12 to 16 inches from the trunk, with a range that depends mainly on the plant's size. As we will see, a tree's energetic essence is concentrated in its trunk, which means we can use its beneficial power better if it is spread out widely across surfaces in the surrounding area.

The Influence of Trees on the Biosphere

Continued research on bioenergetics has revealed another wonderful vital role that trees have in human well-being. Electromagnetic analyses of vegetation-rich environments have shown that, in certain places, trees can alter the bioenergetic quality of the biosphere and interact with people up to a hundred feet away.

This phenomenon occurs frequently and randomly in forests, parks, gardens, and other wooded spaces, provided there are precise interactions between the plant and certain natural carrier waves. The application of this knowledge means we can create bioenergetic parks and gardens, with rest areas that are particularly healthy for the body, or point out within existing green areas the most effective spaces for regenerating and nourishing our health at the energetic level. The conditions that allow us to obtain all this are as follows:

1. the presence of specific natural electromagnetic vectors that function as carrier waves;

2. the correct positioning of plants in relation to these waves;

3. the correct choice and size of the species to be used, or the characteristics of those already in place.

But to better understand how this phenomenon works, we need to better understand the energetic intensifiers and transmitters that make it possible.

Generator Fields, Vital Energy of the Biosphere

In the 1950s and '60s, Walter Kunnen and the German physicists Reinhard Schneider and Paul Schweitzer discovered through the Lecher antenna that, within the multitude of signals that pass through the environment at any moment, there are two fundamental natural carrier waves that are intimately linked to our evolution: they are the large orthogonal and diagonal electromagnetic nets that distribute vital information for humans, animals, and plants into the biosphere. Their origin, although still uncertain, probably depends on the interaction between the earth's rotation and the electromagnetic fields that come from the universe and from inside the earth itself.

We can imagine them as two giant overlapping electromagnetic nets surrounding our planet, each with its own spe-cific frequency, one rotated 45 degrees from the other. Let's try to lay out what these large nets look like in three dimensions.

Their structure is created by the regular and periodic peaks of energy in our environment. Like very soft blades, they vertically cross the entirety of the biosphere, at a slight incline. As the signal moves down from each peak its intensity dimin-ishes, to rise again at the next one.

The large orthogonal net is composed of horizontal en-ergy vectors that run parallel from west to east with 75 feet be-tween them, and cardinal ones that go from north to south with peaks every 100 feet. Seen from above, these vectors cross to form a grid, with squares measuring 75 by 100 feet.

The large diagonal net has a 45-degree incline compared with the cardinal points, with vectors from the northwest and southwest forming squares of 120 feet to the side. The distances between these intervals are approximate, as they are subject to influence by many physical and energetic factors on the earth's surface.

The quality and intensity of the biological information (carried waves) transmitted by the large nets varies from place to place, because they "collect" electromagnetism coming from the cosmos, the sun, and the terrestrial environment, spreading it along their way. Unfortunately the heavy pres-ence of various forms of pollution in our habitat is weaken-ing and transforming the supply of vital energy transmitted by these precious sources of energy, generating forms of chronic fatigue or aggressive biological influences in both plants and humans. The energetic structure of the horizontal, vertical, and northwest vectors is nonetheless such that it plays a central role in bioenergetic landscape technique, and thus these vectors are often called "generator fields." The southwest vector is not used because it usually has levorotatory influences, which can disturb or upset plants. Let's look now at how these electromagnetic fields work together with trees for our well-being.

The Lecher antenna has shown us that when the intensity peak of one of the three generator fields passes through the trunk of a tree, the plant is involved in an exchange of information that has marked effects on the surrounding area. Like a colored lens, the tree can alter the waves carried by the vector as they leave the trunk, coloring them with its specific energetic properties. For example, if the tree in question is a beneficial plant like a linden, we could expect that the carried waves would assume characteristics that are very favorable for the body, despite their qualities upon entering the tree. Thus it is a process of "coloring" that the biological frequencies emitted by the tree apply to those of the signal that passes through it, the same way as if we were to plunge a glass of ink into a clear stream. The difference lies in the fact that, unlike the ink, the tree's energy never runs out.

The cause of this process probably resides in the close dependent relationship that has always existed between plants and the natural energies of the place they are obligated to grow in. But why does this happen in the trunk, rather than a branch? The trunk of a tree is a bit like the neck of a human. It is a channel through which very important circulatory vessels and organic connections pass, which if damaged could stop or do serious harm to biological processes. At the same time, from an energetic perspective, the trunk seems to possess characteristics that are similar to the human torso, which is home to important organs and vital functions.

Active Plants and Bioenergetic Areas

What we have described as a sort of energetic metamorphosis acts on both the bioelectromagnetic intensity and quality of a place, and is measurable across a vast space called the "bioenergetic area." Its geometric formation is not circular around a tree, but extends in the direction of the generator field; it is clearly three-dimensional and has a distinctive elliptical form, similar to an enlarged ovoid with soft edges.

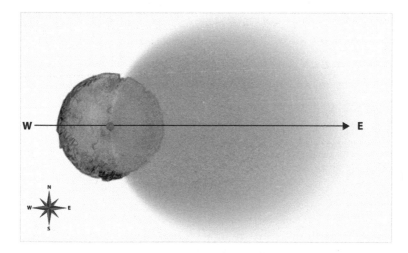

It originates from the center of the trunk and extends in a long parabola up to a 32- to 65-foot distance, weakening in intensity as it moves farther away from the tree. Its shape likely depends on the action caused by the "electromagnetic wind" of the generator field, just as a breeze changes the shape of a cloud.

The electromagnetic thrust of the vector coming from the west thus creates an area toward the east, the thrust of the vector coming from the north creates an area toward the south, and the thrust of the vector coming from the northwest creates an area toward the southeast. At its extremities, the effects weaken much faster and the generator fields regain energetic predominance. This phenomenon happens randomly very frequently in a forest or any space full of trees, which contributes to creating a regenerative atmosphere. If we want to use the bioenergetic landscape to create ideal green spaces for our well-being, it is extremely important to choose "active" plants and position them correctly. The effects produced by one very positive plant, such as an oak, are rather different from those created by a cypress. Both generate this phenomenon, but with opposing values: one is beneficial and the other is harmful. This intervention heavily influences the electromagnetic quality of the local biosphere.

The Energy of Ancient Trees

Some trees have grown in places that are particularly favorable to them. This has made them more resistant to natural adversities and the attacks of humans and animals, so they live longer, even hundreds of years. Much of the credit for this goes to the electromagnetic conditions of the place, particularly the presence of generator fields that are loaded with beneficial influences (at least originally). These areas also provide great bioenergetic areas for us.

Among the many hundreds of possible examples scattered around the world, there are a couple of monumental trees in Italy. The island of Sardinia is home to one of the oldest trees in Europe: the wild olive tree of Luras (in the province of Sassari). It is estimated to be more than 3,000 years old and reaches a height of over 45 feet, and the trunk has a circumference of nearly 60 feet: a true patriarch. Its trunk is crossed through by a powerful northwesterly energetic peak. Its area of bioenergetic influence extends for an astonishing 300-plus feet, with excellent results on many organs, including the immune and circulatory systems, liver, small intestine, colon, and more.

The "Plane tree of 100 soldiers" in Caprino Veronese (province of Verona) dates back to 1370 and is Italy's largest. It is a majestic tree, declared a national monument, with a trunk circumference of 50 feet. The tree has grown in conformity with the peak of a strong east-west vector, creating a huge bioenergetic area that extends eastward more than 260 feet. The biological value is extremely favorable here, too, especially for the lymphatic system, skin, immune system, small intestine, and thyroid.

We should note that all monumental trees, when they interact with generator fields, give rise to remarkably extensive bioenergetic areas, endowing favorable conditions on a vast surrounding area. There are numerous examples of these all around the world, such as the giant sequoias and Douglas firs of North America (*Sequoia sempervirens* and *Pseudotsuga menziesii*), the large ceiba in Central America, the distinctive baobab in Madagascar (*Adansonia grandidieri*), as well as *Eucalyptus regnans* in Australia.

Bioenergetic Areas and Sacred Trees

It is very likely that the oldest traditions connected to the cult of sacred trees and the profound respect for them were based on a sensitivity to these electromagnetic fields and an interpretation of them as a mysterious and thus divine force. Their particular benefit may have been associated with the work of one or more divinities to which the tree or forest was dedicated. Today we can try to interpret the documents of the past, but we will remain unaware of important experiential phenomena. The real visceral and emotional involvement of these phenomena in the life of our ancestors was impossible to communicate in any way other than the language of symbols, magic, and the sacred. For example, in Greek mythology the ash tree was dedicated to Poseidon, god of the sea, springs, and rivers. Bioenergetic analysis of this tree identifies a strong beneficial influence for the kidneys, bladder, and lymphatic system, all of which pertain to the flow of liquids through the body.

Today we know that to stroll through a forest is to be in an environment that is strongly influenced by the bioelectromagnetic properties of trees, so that our excursions in nature are moments of deep energetic therapy. These "sacred" trees and forests are still deserving of the great respect and recognition that we can grant them.

The Bioenergetic Garden: A Sacred Space for Our Health

We can imagine a bioenergetic garden like a silent green concert, where trees and plants are "energy instruments" and the cells in our bodies are mesmerized listeners.

There is something extremely precious about this knowledge, which goes beyond the mere aesthetic value of the landscape. It is based on a sophisticated perceptive listening to the environment that can help us consciously give voice to what ancient cultures called "sacred space," a place where, as Mircca Eliade would say, we feel protected from intrusions from whatever could harm us, where the *genius loci* is manifested in the most positive version of itself. This place of respect can be considered the healing space par excellence.

This explains why it is particularly advisable to create bioenergetic gardens in places that foster relaxation and encourage listening and a calm experience of the environment and our own bodies. We can arrange trees and plants so as to create a sort of "open-air temple" that enhances the therapeutic and energetic power given to us by the plant world, melding it with our own energies. In urban environments, bioenergetic gardens are even more precious, because they pop up in the chaos of everyday life like an island of true electromagnetic recuperation from stress. Ultimately, all we really need is a quiet place, a small tree, and a bench.

The Bioenergetic Landscape and
Its Therapeutic Uses

Knowledge of the potentially beneficial impact of plants on the body and the biosphere opens up new perspectives for supporting and improving our mental and physical health. First and foremost, it offers to everyone the possibility of spending time in restorative natural spaces. Exposure to these spaces is particularly beneficial to those suffering from debilitating conditions. Many experiments confirm that electrosensitive people are able to experience a type of electromagnetic regeneration that allows their bodies to recover faster and more efficiently. This effect is reinforced by the fact that the electromagnetic fields of trees can also protect us from electrosmog. If we hug or otherwise touch a beneficial plant, the effect on our organism is so intense that it wards off the aggressions of the surrounding environment.

This phenomenon occurs on an even larger scale within a bioenergetic area. The quality of the biosphere that is created inside this space is so strong it can neutralize the aggressions or disturbance caused by other signals passing through, like mobile phones or power lines, without throwing the signals off course. In practice, a bioenergetic area doesn't quite act as a shield, but its dextrorotatory biological affinity dominates disruptive electromagnetic fields, keeping our bodies from feeling their effects. Thus we can understand the use of such areas within city parks, where the level of environmental electrosmog is highest.

One recent example of a healing bioenergetic area is the garden in Piazza Vittorio Emanuele II, in Rome, Italy. Created in 1888 at the heart of the Esquiline Hill, this is an area of approximately seven acres at the center of the largest piazza in the city. It also contains some interesting archaeological ruins. The garden, which is very popular with visitors, has many very old trees (planes, Lebanon cedars, magnolias, palms) and rare specimens. A bioenergetic survey was taken in the park and identified thirty perfectly positioned beneficial trees. After measuring the effects of each bioenergetic area on the various organs of the body, a wellness trail was created, with informational signs indicating how to mindfully take in the energy of the various species. Benches were placed in the most beneficial spots to help people improve their health, reduce stress, and sustain vital functioning.

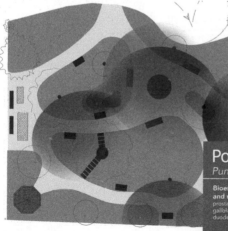

There are other bioenergetic gardens that are open by appointment in several places in Italy, for example, the bio-energetic historic park of the villa Seghetti Panichi in Castel di Lama in Marche (the first of its kind in Italy), the historic Villa Lina garden in Ronciglione (Lazio), and the bioenergetic garden of Castello Quistini in Rovato (Lombardy). The bioenergetic therapeutic garden of Villa Boffo (see previous page) in Biella (Piedmont) is designed to help Alzheimer's sufferers.

Without a doubt, one of the most famous and interesting places to visit is the Bosco del Sorriso (Smile Forest), established in 2012 at the Zegna Oasis in Biella. There is a 1.5-mile path, always open to visitors, that follows a cross-country ski trail through a forest composed mainly of beeches but also home to birches, firs, and larches. The 2011 study identified sixteen trees located at ideal points along the route, each of which creates a bioenergetic area with extremely favorable conditions. A stamp on the trunk allows us to identify the trees, and different signs indicate which organs of the body are most affected, the extent of the trees' influence, and where to position yourself for the most benefit. Thousands of tourists visit the Bosco del Sorriso each year and come away having experienced inner harmony and expanded their awareness of the therapeutic power of nature.

Applying the concepts behind bioenergetic landscapes offers an opportunity for natural therapy in its broadest form, which goes beyond the psychological benefits. A bioenergetic space gives people the opportunity to take as long a break as possible in a space that is able to produce intense effects on their health.

Instruments and Means of Verification

Until now it has not been possible to substitute the simplicity and versatility of the Lecher antenna with electronic instruments for these types of investigations. However, research in the sector of instrumental surveying is always evolving and producing increasingly sensitive tools that are capable of measuring what happens to our bodies under certain conditions. Studies on the bioenergetic landscape have been supported by numerous tests with highly advanced diagnostic devices that can capture even the subtlest variations in human health.

Tests have been conducted by specialists in bioresonance equipment and GDV (Gas Discharge Visualization) bioelectrography instruments developed by Konstantin Korotkov, a professor of computer science and biophysics at Saint Petersburg State University.

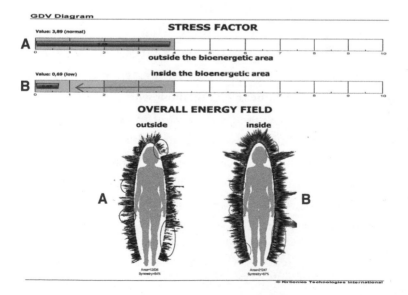

These instruments are used in diagnostic medicine and can show a person's electromagnetic state, obtaining biological information on the state of their health in real time. There have also been numerous technical-instrumental studies in the optic, infraoptic, and vibrational fields using special computerized video cameras equipped with highly sensitive sensors like TRV (a Variable Resonance Camera, which registers emotional or physiological changes) that even from a distance can capture the very weak energy or vibrational fields emitted by humans. One program in particular can translate this data into images that make visible what is usually invisible or simply "felt."

All these new technologies prove the existence of what we call HEFs (human energy fields) and VEFs (vegetable energy fields), and the interaction between them. Verifications have been carried out with these and other tools, both inside and outside beneficial areas, with various types of plants. The results show that inside these areas there is an increase in the complex energetic state of the organism compared with the measurements taken just outside one of these spaces, confirming the existence of areas of influence created by the trees and their real electromagnetic engagement with the human body. The drastic decrease in stress levels after just a few minutes spent in these conditions is astonishing. This effect also occurs when we hug or have physical contact with beneficial trees.

Thanks to these various surveying and verification methods, we can better understand the health benefits that trees and plants have to offer.

What Can We Do for Trees?

Establishing an energy dialogue with the green world enables us to give back with new methods and instruments for improving plant well-being. Of course the most significant act today, for both trees and humans, would be eliminating harmful artificial electromagnetic fields, especially those created by wireless communications (cellular phones, Wi-Fi, etc.). The proliferation of these is creating endless damage to life and the biosphere. Aside from this crucial matter, there are other actions within our reach. For example, various practical experiments in agriculture and new scientific research such as the work of the International Laboratory for Plant Neurobiology in Florence, which shows that to a certain extent plants "love" music, or, rather, certain frequencies and rhythms. Bioenergetic surveys expand the application potential in this sector, allowing us to quickly identify which frequencies are the most effective for favorably stimulating the nervous and immune systems of each botanical species, thus aiding the plant's growth and health and increasing its capacity to respond to pathogenic agents. Another field of application of bioenergetic measurements more specifically addresses plant care—we have seen that nutrition and health are not just about chemistry but also electromagnetism. More effective products are being created in the sector of agricultural and decorative greenery, as we can now identify and choose the most bioactive substances, and avoid the distribution of useless or harmful elements over plants and the soil.

Ultimately, we can safely say the "green thumb" exists.

When we hug trees, they respond to our energy. We can measure and distinguish the reaction of a tree or a simple geranium to our best (or even worst) attentions. New and fascinating experiments and instrumental verifications are under way.

We certainly have a lot more to discover on this topic, but an open mind will help us to emerge from our limited understanding and act with heightened awareness for the universal good.

The Right Place

To benefit from the properties of plants, it's not necessary to have a bioenergetic garden. Just a walk in the woods or a public park to touch or hug a beneficial tree is enough, staying as long as you'd like.

If you want to find a green area that is favorable for your level of energy, having and knowing how to use a Lecher antenna would be ideal, following the aforementioned principles. If this is not possible, and you want to lie in the grass under a tree but don't know whether it's in the "right" place, you can position yourself southeast from the trunk, at a distance no farther than 10 to 20 feet (depending on the size of the tree). This way, even if you don't know whether the tree is crossed by electromagnetic vectors, you'll still have a higher chance of receiving the tree's benefits. Placing yourself in this location to relax or to practice yoga, stretching, or Tai Chi will result in a greater chance of receiving the great bioenergetic gifts of the trees.

After all, the bioenergetic garden is everywhere. You just

need to know how to find it. The respect and gratitude that trees inspire can help us to develop our intuition, which is deeply rooted in our connection with the energies of nature. If we let ourselves, we might even be able to sense a touch of ancient mystery and the sweet, smiling presence of an old "spirit of place."

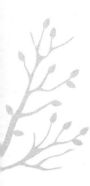

The Air We Breathe

What we call air is a mixture of gases that make up the lowest part of the atmosphere, a vital and dynamic layer known as the troposphere, which is about four-fifths nitrogen and one-fifth oxygen. Small quantities of other gases, fine dust particles, microorganisms, seeds, molecules of water, and carbon dioxide are also present in the troposphere.

Its constant flow in and out of the body during respiration, a process common to all living things, led the ancients to make it one of the four fundamental elements of nature, and even a divinity in some religions. The Egyptian god Shu was the mythical personification of air and cosmic space, while one of the central figures in ancient Vedic texts, Vayu, is the god of wind and air, as well as the divine breath that makes the world live and breathe. Many centuries later, Greek philosopher Anaximenes (c. 586–c. 528 BC) considered air the first matter in the universe and the force that animates living beings.

Yet no matter how high the regard in which it has been held, today it is difficult to find places or environments that can be said to have pure air. The World Health Organization recognizes that air pollution is one of the main environmental risk factors for human health, along with greenhouse gas emissions, global warming, and the impact of climate change. According to their estimates, 90 percent of the world's urban-dwelling population is exposed to harmful levels of air pollution. Combustion processes (transport, heating, industry, and more) continue to be the main source of air pollutants, including particulate matter, sulfur dioxide, benzene, carbon monoxide, and heavy metals (arsenic, cadmium, mercury, and nickel). Other forms of pollution released into the atmosphere by industrial processes and everyday materials can also be added to this list: solvents, volatile organic compounds (VOCs), ammonia, dioxin, furan, polycyclic aromatic compounds (PACs)— the list could go on.

These pollutants cause reactions that are harmful to our health, such as acute respiratory difficulties and chronic illnesses that can lead to death. This is without taking into account the serious damage caused by soil and water pollution. Of course, the concentration of pollutants varies significantly depending on location. Yet wind can spread these substances everywhere, not only from the city to the countryside but also across oceans. It is safe to say that today air pollution is a truly global problem: there is no place on earth where we can breathe truly clean air.

All this carries enormous costs to human health and the environment.

Air in Interior Spaces

According to the World Health Organization, approximately 3 billion people still heat their homes and cook by burning solid fuel such as wood, coal, and crop waste. This is especially true in rural and less-developed parts of the world. Exposure to the fine particles and carbon monoxide released by these fuels into the home causes something like 4.3 million deaths a year, particularly affecting women and children.

While this is happening in less-developed parts of the world, wealthier populations certainly aren't living with different air. Our globalized and industrialized society is now bound by a shared destiny: we spend at least 90 percent of our time in enclosed spaces (home, office, school, health-care facilities, cinemas and theaters, restaurants, etc.), and this number goes up if we add time spent on modes of transport. As a result, we inhale more than 10,000 liters of "spoiled" air every day.

With rare exceptions, in these environments we find a strong presence of materials made up of chemical substances that frequently release volatile or powdery substances. These substances are usually toxic to some extent, are not perceptible by smell, and influence the quality of the air we breathe. Examples of these materials are: upholstery, furniture, paint, and electronic equipment, as well as detergents, cosmetic products, plastic objects (including toys), air fresheners, air purifiers, and so on.

We should add that the air in internal environments is in fact no healthier than the air outside. In fact, it is exactly the same air, plus the emissions produced by materials, our activities, and our very presence.

Living or working by a busy road, where spaces have been recently constructed or restructured with building techniques we erroneously define as "traditional"—in other words, that have been in common use since the sixties and seventies— exposes people to an enormous quantity of volatile and chemical substances and microparticles. And superficial attention paid to the environment hardly helps. According to chemist Hermann Fischer, a pioneer in the natural paint industry, "water-based" or acrylic paints are falsely ecological because they contain hundreds of chemical substances, including additives and cosolvents, which are seriously harmful to the environment. Some of these toxic ingredients (like formaldehyde, ammonia, and white spirit) emit fumes into the air over the course of many years, accumulating in the internal environment. The same goes for glues, synthetic flooring, plaster with chemical additives, sealers and finishes for wood and metal, and textiles, including natural fabrics that are treated with other substances.

We do have other options—the techniques and materials used in bioconstruction, if used correctly, are invaluable. Bioconstruction improves comfort and avoids the use of these substances, thus minimizing the disasters that ordinary building causes not just for our habitat but the entire planet. Shifting to bioconstruction is more urgent than ever. One only has to consider that in enclosed spaces the presence of the aforementioned VOCs can reach concentrations 10 or 20 times higher than in the outdoors, and more than 350 different types of them have been detected. The most common VOCs of synthetic origin are formaldehyde, considered by many the most prominent pollutant in our homes (and which is indeed an ingredient in many glues, paints, cladding panels, fabrics, and more); benzene (found in plastics, resins, synthetic fibers, and tobacco smoke); perchloroethylene and tetrachloroethylene (used in dry cleaning); acetone and other solvents; hydrocarbons; compounds containing chlorine; and many others.

Pollution from VOCs is a global problem and the main cause of the sick building syndrome (SBS) and building-related illness (BRI), the symptions of which can be general illnesses, headaches, irritation of the eyes and throat, nausea, respiratory problems, loss of concentration, and even asthma and allergies. It is no coincidence that these ailments have become particularly common since the seventies, particularly in new buildings.

The materials and machinery used in construction frequently cause physical pollution. The synthetic mineral fibers often used for thermal and sound insulation, such as mineral wool, fiberglass, or microfibers, are easily pulverized and therefore easily breathable. In recent years nanoparticles of various materials have been found in the air inside buildings, so small they can pass through the cellular membrane. The effects of these on humans are still unknown.

In enclosed spaces, varying levels of biological and microbiological pollution also occur, in the form of molds, bacteria, and viruses. The concentration of this pollution is often linked to the presence of people and pets. Bedrooms are frequently full of these pollutants. Molds that we can see on the walls, for example, are just the most obvious aspect of their proliferation in our interior surroundings (which occur most prevalently in mattresses, clothing, wardrobes, etc.), often resulting from a combination of poor humidity management, like laundry hung to dry and moisture coming from bathrooms, and insufficient wall insulation. This also feeds the proliferation of mites, whose droppings most people are allergic to.

Furthermore, a significant quantity of bioeffluents are found in enclosed spaces. These are a group of more than 150 substances produced by humans and pets through respiration, perspiration, and other normal biological functions. Indeed, while we are indoors, we emit waste substances such as carbon dioxide, water vapor, ethanol, acetone, methanol, and acetic ether.

Good ventilation of spaces is fundamental to reducing the concentration of humidity and polluting agents in the air, especially in very crowded or warm spaces. But often it is not practiced as required, especially in very energy-efficient buildings or where the air is forcibly introduced or conditioned, such as in offices, banks, and hospitals. Air-conditioning equipment, among other things, can play host to harmful microorganisms. In 1976, 34 veterans of the American Legion died from an illness caused by bacteria, then called *Legionella*, present in the air-conditioning of the hotel they were staying in.

Sometimes we avoid ventilating our homes properly with the excuse of the climate or bothersome external elements such as traffic or noise, but we must never forget that poor air circulation often causes significant accumulations of very aggressive substances like formaldehyde and fine particles. Even if we can't see the air pollution in a space, it may still make us feel unwell.

It is important to add that forced-air systems, synthetic materials, and electromagnetic and electrostatic fields dramatically reduce the concentration of small negative ions, which, according to some scientists, are the true source of air vitality. The enclosed spaces we spend most of our time in are not always the right places to breathe fully and deeply.

Respiration, Photosynthesis, Transpiration

The air and everything it is made up of are at the center of the respiratory process, which is a metabolic function intended to produce energy in living beings through an exchange of gases between the organism and its external environment. The mechanisms of this process, however, differ between animals and plants.

On a macroscopic level, human beings and other mammals breathe by actively inhaling air through the lungs that contains oxygen, which is transported by the blood to all the organs and tissues in the body. Then we expel air enriched with carbon dioxide (CO_2). Of the air that we breathe in, oxygen makes up 21 percent and carbon dioxide 0.03 percent (in 2015 this value was updated to 0.04 percent). Of the air that we breathe out, however, oxygen makes up only 16 percent, while carbon dioxide goes up to 5 percent. This process involves a series of chemical reactions at the cellular level, in which oxygen is consumed and heat, carbon dioxide, and water are produced. As a result, when we breathe, perspiration takes place, which is the release of water vapor.

Plants also need oxygen and are always respiring, but the process takes place passively and involves all their cells. Even the roots absorb oxygen through the water and air in the earth. In plants, respiration serves the purpose of releasing the energy contained in the sugars and other substances produced and accumulated during photosynthesis, making them available for the growth and vital activities of the organism. During this activity, oxygen is consumed and carbon dioxide and water vapor are produced. The latter are then dispersed into the atmosphere through the leaves.

Plants are able to capture and store the energy of the sun through photosynthesis (from the Greek *photo*, light, and *synthesis*, construction), converting it into chemical energy. This function allows the plant to independently produce the sugars that constitute its nutrition and source of energy. In the majority of plants, photosynthesis takes place within organelles called chloroplasts, found in the leaves and other green parts. Chloroplasts are rich in chlorophyll and other light-sensitive pigments. The phenomenon takes place during the day when there is sunlight, separating the water absorbed by the roots into hydrogen and oxygen. The plants absorb carbon dioxide, which combines with the hydrogen to produce glucose and oxygen, a gas that is then released into the surroundings. The majority of the oxygen present in the earth's atmosphere is indeed produced by plants (including algae), which currently make up around 99.5 percent of the planet's biomass. This is an enormous percentage when we consider that humans and all other living things make up less than 0.5 percent. At the same time, photosynthesis consumes around 25 times more carbon dioxide than the amount consumed through respiration, a ratio that is clearly to the benefit of the other inhabitants of Earth.

Iain Stewart, a professor at Plymouth University, confirmed this in an experiment. In September 2011 he survived for two days in an airtight, 120-square-foot chamber made of transparent Plexiglas and filled with more than 150 plants at the Eden Project's Rainforest Biome in Cornwall. The initial levels of oxygen were relatively low, around 12.5 percent (as at high altitude), causing him to experience several negative symptoms, but after a few hours photosynthesis brought the levels up to 21 percent, the same as at sea level, showing that it is possible to survive on the oxygen produced by plants alone.

The passage of gases and water vapor between the interior and exterior of the plant is controlled by stomata. Stomata are small pores usually found on the underside of leaves, and how much they open is regulated by the environmental conditions and the needs of the plant. The stomata also regulate the plant's water content through transpiration, a circular process by which water and minerals are taken up through the roots to be released from the leaves and stems as water vapor. This produces an interesting phenomenon: the tissues of the leaves cool down, creating a downward convection of air. The air then enters into contact with the earth and the rhizosphere, a miniature universe made up of roots and huge quantities of microorganisms that work to break down and transform useful substances and volatile pollutants into nourishment and energy.

Plants, in turn, take great care of their root microorganisms, as they release up to 45 percent of the substances produced through photosynthesis into the rhizosphere. This is the most obvious explanation for why houseplants are generally capable of removing volatile pollutants from enclosed spaces.

Purify the Air and Improve the Environment with Plants

If the main causes of poor air quality in enclosed spaces are the hermetic insulation of buildings, the synthetic materials used, bioeffluents, and reduced ventilation, it would be hard to think of anything worse than a space shuttle.

Back in 1973, NASA scientists realized that the quality of air inside the Skylab space station, loaded with at least 107 volatile organic compounds, was creating serious problems for its occupants. Given that it was impossible to change the materials and technologies used in these spaces, in the 1980s Bill Wolverton ran some experiments at NASA's John C. Stennis Space Center. The findings revealed that the presence of certain indoor plants could reduce levels of formaldehyde, benzene, trichloroethylene, and many other VOCs and pollutants in the air. The first biohome project, which was a hermetically sealed experimental living facility made from completely synthetic materials, provided for the purification not only of the inside air but also of water. Water was purified through aspiration and mechanical pumping toward the roots of a plant system made up of various types of plants (the filtering capability exponentially increased with the variety). Wolverton's studies allowed us to understand the mechanisms by which plants, through transpiration, draw contaminated toxic air to their roots and turn it into food. He identified 50 houseplants that are capable of purifying the main volatile pollutants from the air, regulating humidity, and creating vital oxygen. In order of overall efficacy:

Areca palm (*Chrysalidocarpus lutescens*)

Rhapis (*Rhapis excelsa*)

Bamboo palm (*Chamaedorea seifrizii*)

Ficus (*Ficus robusta* or *elastica*)

Janet Craig dracaena (*Dracaena deremensis* "Janet Craig")

Ivy (*Hedera helix*)

Dwarf date palm (*Phoenix roebelenii*)

Ficus alii (*Ficus maclellandii* "Alii")

Boston fern (*Nephrolepis exaltata* "Bostoniensis")

Peace lily (*Spathiphyllum*)

Massangeana dracaena (*Dracaena fragrans* "Massangeana")

Pothos aureus (*Epipremnum aureum* or *Scindapsus aureus*)

Kimberley queen fern (*Nephrolepis obliterata*)

Chrysanthemum (*Chrysanthemum morifolium*)

Gerbera (*Gerbera jamesonii*)

Warneckei dracaena (*Dracaena deremensis* "Warneckei")

Dragon tree (*Dracaena marginata*)

Blushing philodendron (*Philodendron erubescens*)

Arrowhead plant (*Syngonium podophyllum*)

Exotica compacta dieffenbachia (*Dieffenbachia* "Exotica Compacta")

Parlor palm (*Chamaedorea elegans*)

Benjamin fig (*Ficus benjamina*)

Dwarf umbrella tree (*Schefflera arboricola*)

Begonia (*Begonia semperflorens*)

Lacy tree philodendron (*Philodendron selloum*)

Heartleaf philodendron (*Philodendron scandens*)

Snake plant (*Sansevieria trifasciata*)

Dumb cane (*Dieffenbachia camilla*)

Elephant philodendron (*Philodendron domesticum*)

Norfolk pine (*Araucaria heterophylla*)

Homalomena (*Homalomena wallisii*)

Prayer plant (*Maranta leuconeura* "Kerchoveana")

Dwarf banana (*Musa cavendishii*)

Epiphilum or Christmas cactus (*Schlumbergera bridgesii* or *Schlumbergera rhipsalidopsis*)

Grape ivy (*Cissus rhombifolia*)

Lilyturf (*Liriope spicata*)

Orchid (*Dendrobium*)

Spider plant (*Chlorophytum comosum* "Vittatum")

Silver Queen (*Aglaonema crispum* "Silver Queen")

Flamingo flower (*Anthurium andaeanum*)

Garden croton (*Codiaeum variegatum pictum*)

Poinsettia (*Euphorbia pulcherrima*)

Dwarf azalea (*Rhododendron simsii* "Compacta")

Peacock plant (*Calathea makoyana*)

Aloe vera (*Aloe barbadensis*)

Cyclamen (*Cyclamen persicum*)

Urn plant (*Aechmea fasciata*)

Tulip (*Tulipa gesneriana*)

Sander's moth orchid (*Phalaenopsis sanderiana, Phalaenopsis* spp.)

Kalanchoe (*Kalanchoe blossfeldiana*)

Subsequent research has added knowledge of the plants' ability to absorb airborne pollutant particles and to reduce positive ions and produce negative ions, which—as we have seen—brings innumerable benefits. Since then, there has been great interest in better understanding the mechanisms by which these plants carry out the purification processes. A German study published in 1994 in the *Plant Physiology Journal* examined the ability of the leaves of a chlorophytum, or spider plant (*Chlorophytum comosum*), to absorb or destroy some chemical compounds. The researchers exposed only the leafy part to formaldehyde with radioactive carbon 14, and showed that the substance can be effectively assimilated and converted into plant tissue and other substances that are useful to the plant.

The decomposition of pollutants by microbes living around the plant's roots has also been studied. In some research, these microbes appear to be better than the leaves at absorbing harmful volatile substances like formaldehyde. It is commonly thought that these microbes, along with oxygen, feed the colonies of bacteria that live in the root area, making them increasingly efficient at purification, and even more effective when the concentration of pollutants is higher.

Ronald Wood and Margaret Burchett of the University of Technology Sydney have devoted themselves to furthering knowledge of the VOC purification process carried out synergically by indoor plants and by microorganisms that live in contact with their roots. According to the researchers, potted plants constitute a self-regulating microcosm. They are able to carry out the botanical purification (which Wood and Burchett have named "phytoremediation") of air quality and cleanliness in enclosed spaces, by activating a complex process of biofiltration.

It is even easier to understand the phenomenon when we

see that the majority of indoor plants belong to species that originate from tropical rainforests, where they live in a hot and humid climate at the base of much taller plants. Therefore they receive little direct sunlight and share their rhizosphere with a huge number of colonies of microorganisms that are highly specialized for carrying out the various tasks of digestion of and transformation into substances that are useful to the plant.

Many other research projects have been carried out in closed control chambers, into which precise percentages of pollutants are introduced at the start, and after some hours with the plants, their concentration is measured. However, in non-laboratory situations, there is a constant release of volatile pollutants and a more complex environment. In order to dissipate doubts about the purifying ability of plants, researchers started to propose experiments and measurements that would be carried out in contexts that were more true to life. One of these was conducted inside the offices of a big multinational company in Edinburgh. In the rooms that housed plants, the occupants reported feeling more productive and less oppressed, and enjoyed increased levels of comfort and privacy. A perceptible decrease in short-term absenteeism for health reasons was also observed. The people who worked in the control environments with no plants, however, realized how disadvantaged their conditions were and expressed the desire to have plants in their spaces, too. Who could blame them?

This study and others carried out in real-life environments shared the conclusion that the presence of plants reduces illness and stress and changes people's perceptions of their place of work, increasing comfort, satisfaction, and performance.

These effects are increased further still if the windows open onto green spaces.

It is clear, then, that the benefits of plants in enclosed spaces go far beyond their purifying function, and confirm our innate and "neurological" need for nature.

This is one of the reasons that it so effective to have a variety of plant types, shapes, and sizes in indoor spaces, creating as rich and complex a space as possible. On one hand, this has profound effects on our psychoemotional state, and on the other it increases the synergy and filtering ability of each plant organism, as each species has a particular ability to absorb and break down certain volatile substances.

Plants at Work: The Green Office

In the same way that factors such as the position, visibility, and compositional attractiveness of plants indoors can play a significant psychophysiological role, flowers also have an impact on our senses and mood. For example, bringing them into hospitals has been shown to accelerate the recovery process and reduce the need for drugs, as well as improving people's perceptions of the hospital environment. Furthermore, when tested, it was revealed that if a worker saw a vase of roses on the desk in his or her office, in just four minutes significant psychological and physiological relaxation was felt. It is no surprise that giving someone a bouquet of flowers always makes an impression: they are, perhaps, the quintessence of nature.

The effect of the presence of plants and flowers in the workplace is being studied further in real-life environments, in a quest for proof of its effect on employee well-being as well as on productivity. Compared with the presence of sculptures or the absence of any type of decoration, people react to the addition of botanical elements in their offices with a considerable increase in new ideas. This is the case especially among men, while women have proved to become more creative and flexible.

This debunks the myth subscribed to by proponents of "lean offices" that plants are neither useful nor necessary in working spaces. These are bare, basic spaces inspired by minimalist design. However, if we understand attractiveness and functionality to be the foundations of a high-quality workplace, the results of these studies should persuade open-minded, forward-thinking, and entrepreneurial people to consider greenery in offices as a productive investment.

The proof of its worth comes from a well-known study conducted under real-life conditions in the commercial offices of large companies in the United Kingdom and the Netherlands. The research involved various academic institutions, such as the Universities of Cardiff and Exeter in the UK, Groningen in the Netherlands, and Queensland in Australia, and compares the effects of "lean office" environments on workers with those of offices to which a diverse range of plants have been introduced ("green offices"). In the latter, significant increases were measured in the parameters under study, such as workplace satisfaction (40 percent increase), concentration levels, and perception of air quality. Thus it is proved that plants in "green offices" improve employees' physical, cognitive, and emotional involvement, generating greater happiness and well-being and nurturing a feeling of being cared for by their superiors. It also brings concrete long-term benefits, not least financially. For example, studies showed an increase of up to 15 percent in productivity, which should interest companies. Now new strategies are needed for turning lean offices into green offices. Alex Haslam, a professor at the University of Queensland's School of Psychology and coauthor of the study, commented that the "lean" philosophy has many supporters who are convinced that "less is more," but their research shows that in some respects, "less is just less."

How Much Green Do We Need?

In 2004, the European Union supported an informational campaign called "A little healthy green in the workplace" aimed at encouraging companies and administrators to put plants in offices and all indoor spaces to improve working conditions and help resolve various health issues. The campaign suggested a secure return on the investment. Based on the expectation that companies would provide at least one potted plant per employee, and that sick days would be reduced by at least 1 percent (which equates to a savings of about 30,000 euros a year), for a company of 100 employees the investment would be returned in under 12 months.

So if it is common knowledge that plants bring unquestionable benefits to the quality of the spaces in which we live and work, how do we select and use them in the best way possible? Despite the plethora of studies carried out over the years, we are still lacking precise directions and rules for use. It is almost impossible to accurately cite the numbers and types of plants that can be used in various situations. There are so many variables at play in these evaluations: the type of space, the presence and impact of people, the quantity and quality of natural light, the features of the materials used in the furnishings and surfaces, the possible pollutants that are present, the type and duration of the natural or artificial ventilation, and the quality of the air that is coming in from outside. If then we also want to create environments that "work" on a psychoemotional level, we should introduce enough plants to create a real sense of nature, which has a significant neurological and behavioral impact. Thus, without creating either a rainforest or a sad display of lonely pots, we can determine what certain arrangements will do for our health and our state of mind and proceed accordingly.

The studies carried out in real-life small- or medium-size workplaces suggest that we should have at least one medium-size plant close to the place where we spend the longest amount of time, in order to improve what Wolverton calls the "personal breathing zone." It has been shown that the addition of at least three medium-size plants, such as the *Dracaena deremensis* "Janet Craig", or six small table plants, like peace lilies, effectively removes VOCs from the room.

Kamal Meattle, a New Delhi entrepreneur, provides an example of the application of this idea in an environment that is critically polluted. New Delhi has the highest levels of air pollution in the world. In his company, 300 people work in an area of 15,000 square meters, and they have more than 1,500 plants. Meattle, worried about his health because of smog, read the studies conducted by NASA and others, and decided to introduce three types of low-maintenance purifying plants into his company offices: areca palm (*Chrysalidocarpus lutescens*), snake plant (*Sansevieria trifasciata*), and pothos (*Epipremnum aureum*). The air entering from outside, full of particulate matter, is first "washed," then passes through a greenhouse of more than 400 plants arranged on the roof of the building to remove form-aldehyde, benzene, and carbon monoxide, and finally passes through an antibacterial filter before reaching the work space. Whatever detractors and skeptics may say about the purifying function of plants, many—including the Indian government— recognize Meattle's efforts to produce clean air and a pleasant environment, which yields concrete results in terms of em-ployee health and productivity. Not to mention energy savings of 15 percent, thanks to the reduced need for refreshing the air in the building. Based on his success, for purification and oxygenation of the air, Meattle suggests having at least four shoulder-height areca plants and an average of six to eight san-sevieria and pothos plants per head.

Having considered the various viewpoints and studies on the subject, as well as our own personal experience, we believe that three medium-high plants (for example, dracaena, areca, kentia, or rhapis) will yield good results in terms of purifica-tion, humidification, oxygenation, and ionization in a room of up to 2,500 cubic feet occupied by one person for a significant number of hours (such as an office). You'll want to make sure there is sufficient surface area of soil in the pot and a leaf mass of at least 350 grams.

To get even better results, one or more of these plants should be placed in close proximity to your area of work or study. Of course, the more plants and variety within the plants, the more benefits to the environment, making it an even more pleasant and productive place to be.

Which Plants for Home and Which for the Office?

In the years following Wolverton's early research, many studies expanded the horizon of knowledge on the subject and demonstrated that environmental purification was an ability shared by many indoor plants.

One U.S. study analyzed the efficiency of the leaf surface of 28 houseplants in the removal of 5 types of VOC inside sealed containers: benzene, toluene, trichloroethylene, octane, and alpha-pinene. Red ivy (*Hemigraphis alternata*), common ivy (*Hedera helix*), wax plant (*Hoya carnosa*), and asparagus fern (*Asparagus densiflorus*) were reported to have the highest efficiency with all the pollutants. Purple secretia (*Tradescantia pallida*) was effective on four of them, nerve plant (*Fittonia argyroneura*) effectively removed three, Benjamin ficus (*Ficus benjamina*) two, and ming aralia (*Polyscias fruticosa*) just one. So the effectiveness of the plants varies, and it is becoming more and more evident that synergy is necessary for optimum removal of pollutants.

Vadoud Niri, a researcher at State University of New York at Oswego, recently conducted an experiment in a sealed chamber where he tested the capability of five houseplants to remove eight common volatile organic substances. The plants used were crassulas (*Crassula argentea* or *Crassula ovata*), spider plants (*Chlorophytum comosum*), scarlet stars (*Guzmania ligulata*), Caribbean tree cactus (*Consolea falcata*), and dracaena (*Dracaena fragrans*). In a report presented in August 2016 to the American Chemical Society, Niri describes how some of the plants demonstrated specific abilities to remove certain substances. The scarlet star, a bromeliad, removed more than 80 percent of six of the eight substances in twelve hours. All the plants were effective at removing acetone, but the dracaena was the best, removing 94 percent of the substance. The crassula worked well for toluene, while the spider plant was the fastest to activate the purification process.

This research further confirms that plants vary in their filtering abilities, having been analyzed both in control chambers and in real-life environments. Other specific abilities of each plant are still under study and perhaps difficult to define, specifically because part of the purification is done by the root microorganisms and part by the leaves. The genus *Tillandsia* represents a rather curious exception. Tillandsia are epiphyte plants of mainly tropical origin that do not have underground roots and absorb moisture and nutrients through special openings on their leaves. Research carried out at the University of Florence and University of Bologna demonstrated that some of these plants (for example, *Tillandsia bulbosa*) are very effective at capturing fine dust particulates polluted by hydrocarbons from gas and diesel combustion, and can also metabolize them.

As more research is being conducted, we can look at the specific purposes of certain plants, while bearing in mind that there are no fixed rules, just choices motivated by several variables. All indoor plants are suitable for both the home and the office.

As we mentioned previously, formaldehyde is perhaps the most common pollutant found in the home, but it is even more common in offices. The dangers it poses have been attested to repeatedly, and the European Union has declared that it "may cause cancer" (EU regulation no. 605/2014). It is found in resins, foam insulation, wood glue, paper towels, toilet paper, new fabrics, dyes, carpets, and various adhesives. These are all materials that are used particularly in offices and commercial buildings. From the 50 plants he analyzed, Wolverton compiled a list of the plants that were most efficient in absorbing this pollutant. The list includes the Boston fern and the Kimberley queen fern, followed by chrysanthemum, gerbera, various types of palm (*Phoenix roebelenii, Chamaedorea seifrizii, Areca palmata* or *Chrysalidocarpus lutescens,* and *Rhapis excelsa*), Janet Craig dracaena and Massangeana dracaena, some ficuses (*alii, benjamina,* and *robusta*), spathiphyllum, ivy, and schefflera.

The best plant against ammonia is rhapis (*excelsa*), followed by homalomena, liriope, anthurium, calathea, and dendrobium. Xylene and toluene are removed most effectively by the areca palm and pygmy date palm (*Phoenix roebelenii*), the phalaenopsis orchid, dieffenbachia, and dracaenas. The peace lily (*Spathiphyllum*) deserves a special mention. It is a decorative plant that is very easy to care for, and according to various researchers it has many useful properties. Wolverton considers it a highly effective plant for removing acetone, methanol, and ethanol from the air. These are the main constituents of human bioeffluents. It is also very active against benzene, ammonia, and trichloroethylene.

Tall, compact plants (for example, the Janet Craig dracaena, rhapis and other palms, ficus, etc.) are the best choice for open-plan office spaces. This is to increase the surface area of leaves per square foot. Vines like ivies and chlorophytum can also be hung in baskets. This creates a positive visual as well as greater individual privacy. In fact, in some cases a sort of botanical screen can be created around each workstation that can reduce ambient noise by up to five decibels, create an ideal percentage of humidity in the air, and foster negative ionization.

These solutions naturally work just as well in the home. The bathroom and kitchen are often the spaces with the highest concentration of volatile pollutants and very high levels of humidity. The most versatile and effective plants to use in these spaces, partly because they do not need too much light, are ivy, spider plants, golden pothos, green pothos, and ferns.

As for the bedroom, there is a common opinion that it should not have plants because they consume oxygen and increase humidity, but this is completely false. The amount of carbon dioxide that plants give off during the night is insignificant compared with the amount we expel by breathing, and their presence—even in large quantities—has no bearing on the quality of air. Otherwise, anyone who went camping in the woods for a night would be done for!

Meanwhile, some houseplants have actually earned the reputation (for good reason) of adapting to sleep environments, as they absorb carbon dioxide and release oxygen during the night. The best plants for this purpose are snake plants (*Sansevieria trifasciata*), crassulas, kalanchoes, cactuses (*Epiphyllum*, for example), aloe vera, orchids, and some tillandsia (like *Tillandsia usneoides*). These plants share a special feature: they use CAM (crassulacean acid metabolism) photosynthesis. This is a kind of "two-part" photosynthesis common in plant species that naturally live in dry environments. Their stomata only open during the night to absorb and accumulate carbon dioxide, and in the daytime, during the process of photosynthesis to store the oxygen that will be released during the night, the stomata remain closed to reduce water loss through transpiration. Like all plants, they respire continuously to convert sugars into energy, consuming part of the oxygen produced in photosynthesis.

In terms of humidity, it is thought that while sleeping the average person produces around 500 to 600 grams of water vapor through breathing. Plant transpiration releases around 90 percent of the water absorbed, but the plants mentioned above absorb such a tiny amount of water that nocturnal emission of vapor is negligible. While it is enjoyable and useful to indulge in buying plants for the home and the office, we must be careful in certain settings, such as nursing homes, hospitals, schools, and so on. Some plants are toxic for humans and pets. Many species are poisonous to varying degrees: you cannot ingest the aerial parts of some plants, while in others you shouldn't even touch the sap (dieffenbachia, philodendron, poinsettia, anthurium, *Ficus elastica*, zamioculcas, and in part also spathiphyllum). This characteristic probably comes from the fact that in the undergrowth of their natural environment they had to develop particular features to discourage animals from eating them, so they created poisons that are found in their roots, stems, leaves, and flowers.

There are some general rules that apply to all plants: always keep the leaves clean in order to avoid suffocating the stomata, and respect their need for light, water, care, and nutrients, because they cannot obtain them without our help. If plants are healthy and live in an appropriate environment, they can "work" for us more efficiently. We can also facilitate their purifying abilities by feeding the colonies of root microorganisms with natural fertilizer or by introducing mycorrhizae and polyvalent microbial groups such as "effective microorganisms" (EM), which are becoming increasingly well known for their various uses.

The Bioenergetic Landscape Indoors

Applying this technique in indoor spaces offers an invaluable opportunity to improve, in terms of electromagnetism, the spaces where we spend much of our time. It is especially useful in workplaces and health-care sites, where people are often stressed and exposed to high concentrations of electric and magnetic fields generated by various types of machinery for extended periods. People who are electrosensitive particularly feel the effects of electrosmog, but anyone can benefit from spending time in indoor spaces of energy restoration. Applying the bioenergetic technique, however, is restricted by the size of these spaces, the distinctive traits that electromagnetic fields have in enclosed spaces, and limitations when it comes to choosing ideal plants. The health-boosting areas created might be much smaller than anything that could be made outdoors, but they can certainly work well in large interior spaces.

For example, we have found that in large open-plan offices, just one plant less than six feet tall, if correctly positioned, can have positive effects on up to twelve workstations, spread out in an area of several dozen square feet; this is also true for a doctor's waiting room, the seating area of a large living room, or a spa. Yet only certain houseplants possess the right characteristics for this type of use. To foster a bioenergetic reaction, plant specimens must be sufficiently tall and robust, with a stem of at least one and a half centimeters in diameter or a very dense mass. But, most important, they must be beneficial!

Only a few of the purifying plants indicated in NASA's research conform to these requirements, in part because many of them are poisonous to some extent and this can affect their energetic properties. Palms, dracaenas, ferns, and the indoor dwarf banana tree (*Musa cavendishii*) are perfect. Yet we must exclude others that are usually used for their aesthetic value, such as the ficus (*alii, benjamina, elastica,* and others), as they have properties that are bioelectromagnetically disruptive. Nevertheless, it is useful to note that we can use all medium or small plants everywhere without any problems. It would be wise, though, to place the most voluminous ones that contain toxic substances a few feet away.

Green Offices, Green Buildings

In recent decades, there have been a growing number of proposals for green building initiatives that offer total (rather than partial) solutions in terms of energy saving and improving the quality of our habitats. The types of buildings involved are supplied with enhanced natural ventilation, higher amounts of natural light, and adaptations of the materials and technologies used in order to minimize the building's total environmental impact. These solutions have undeniable advantages. In comparison to more conventionally built environments, the studies report notable increases in comfort, people's perception of their health and appreciation of their workplace, higher levels of productivity, and a reduction of up to 79 percent of the energy used for air-conditioning.

One study conducted at Harvard University demonstrated that employees working in a green building can achieve an increase in cognitive performance of up to 101 percent compared with their performance in a conventional building. This increase has been linked to better ventilation and the consequent reduction in CO_2, in part thanks to the use of low-emission materials. These results were seconded by the U.S. Department of Energy's Lawrence Berkeley National Laboratory, which showed how modest increases in carbon dioxide in study and work spaces can seriously compromise a person's mental performance and decision-making ability. Human respiration, the density of occupants in a space, and most of all, limited or unsuitable ventilation all contribute to increasing the concentration of CO_2, and thus a gradual reduction in performance.

Yet the main objectives of green building initiatives are often technically focused on saving energy and consuming fewer resources, and not always on fulfilling deep human needs, such as our need for more nature. But with the introduction of indoor plants and botanical systems that serve a purpose that is not merely decorative, significant improvements in mood and positive feelings about the workplace have been observed. A 2015 study showed that when presented with several office solutions proposed by architects and designers, the top preference of those surveyed was a large amount of natural light, followed close behind by the presence of plants in the workplace.

The number of options available for introducing plants into offices and other indoor spaces has grown exponentially in recent years. By now everyone has seen the walls of greenery made with plants woven into a support structure, or new ideas for integrating plants into architecture ("vegetecture") or mechanical air biofilter systems activated by purifying plants. It is important to understand how exactly to use plants to improve the livability of our homes and workplaces. If our goal is to make these environments healthier, our first move should be to try to fight the primary causes of dissatisfaction and distress. Experience has shown us that the environments we live in, even those designed according to good principles, are often full of disruptive elements.

Take your average workstation, for example. Desks are often overloaded with high-frequency electromagnetic fields (electric and magnetic fields emanate from cables and equipment, Wi-Fi, cordless phones, etc.), which expose the person using the desk to considerable levels of electrosmog and reduce negative ionization. In this case, contrary to popular belief, plants that are praised for their capacity to absorb electromagnetic waves (such as cacti or tillandsia) are of no use.

The fluorescent lamps used for artificial light also have electronic components that give off radio frequencies, and the spectrum of light they emit is often unbalanced. We spend a long time in spaces like this and the exposure is constant. It is possible to reduce the electromagnetic fields in these environments by taking various precautions both during the planning phase and once the space is already in use. These precautions allow us to limit mental and physical fatigue and to influence the long-term state of health of those exposed to them. Lighting choices should be carefully considered not only in terms of performance but also in terms of eye comfort, which, after all, is directly related to mental comfort.

To improve indoor air quality and general comfort we should also remember the great importance of finishing materials such as paint, plaster, and laminates. And let's not forget cleaning products, which are often of synthetic origin and release enormous quantities of VOCs and all sorts of toxic substances. You can avoid this air pollution by making greener choices and buying all-natural products. Photocatalytic paint can also be useful in some cases—this type of paint removes certain volatile pollutants and particulate matter from the air by oxidizing and transforming them into harmless elements, similar to the way plants purify the environment.

Improving the quality of the spaces in which we live and work is not only an expression of sensitivity but also of respect for life. Humans risk losing their instinctive and animal nature by passively yielding to technology and habit. But our body's intelligence, with its perceptions and needs, will win out. Understanding the special contribution that plants make to our habitat gives us a chance to awaken our consciousness and helps us appreciate the presence of plants and take care of them, not just because they are useful but also because we are all part of a single, immense living organism.

There are truly so many ways to benefit from nature's great therapeutic power. Integrating the different techniques described in this book is an effective way to expand the quality and quantity of our interaction with natural environments. This new research makes it possible to surpass the narrow and antiquated symptom-cure model offered by other ways of approaching the issue of health, especially in relation to the lifestyles that are on the rise in our society. We all know that nature knows us (and recognizes us) as complete beings, children of our shared environment and the product of our own evolution. Its response to our need for well-being will be all the greater the more we can consciously express this need. We hope this book can help to broaden this awareness.

One last thing: a few days ago, as we were going down a

road we don't usually take at sunset, some trees (common linden trees—*Tilia americana*) spoke to us.

What did they say? Well, it's obvious: what we have been whispering for ages, forever, with patient benevolence:

sometimes trees persist
closer to you
than you had thought

they emerge

even the darkest
bear light
a sudden dark reassurance

(JOHN TAYLOR, "BUT IT WAS NOT YET NIGHT")

We reflected a little, as we listened . . .
And then, overcome with affection, we gave them a hug.

1: Nature's Imprint: Is It Truly Forever?

J. D. Balling, J. H. Falk, "Development of Visual Preference for Natural Environments," *Environment and Behavior* 14(1), 1982: 5–28.

B. De Coensel et al., "Effects of Natural Sounds on the Perception of Road Traffic Noise," *Journal of Acoustical Society of America* 129(4), 2011: 148–53.

V. Lobue, J. S. Deloache, "Superior Detection of Threat-relevant Stimuli in Infancy," *Developmental Science* 13(1), 2010: 221–28.

J. New et al., "Category-Specific Attention for Animals Reflects Ancestral Priorities, Not Expertise," *Proceedings of the National Academy of Sciences of the United States of America* 104(16), 2007: 598–603.

D. Sadava et al., "L'evoluzione della specie umana," in *La nuova biologia.blu* (Bologna: Zanichelli, 2016).

R. S. Ulrich, "Visual Landscapes and Psychological Well-being," *Landscape Research* 4, 1979: 17–23.

R. S. Ulrich et al., "Stress Recovery During Exposure to Natural and Urban Environments," *Journal of Environmental Psychology* 11, 1991: 201–30.

R. S. Ulrich et al., "Effects of Exposure to Nature and Abstract Pictures on Patients Recovering from Open Heart Surgery," *Journal of Society for Psychophysiological Research* 30 (suppl. 1), 1993: 7.

E. O. Wilson, *Biophilia: The Human Bond with Other Species* (Cambridge, MA: Harvard University Press, 1984).

E. O. Wilson, *The Future of Life* (New York: Knopf, 2002).

Worldwatch Institute, *State of the World 2007: Our Urban Future* (New York: Norton, 2007).

2: Is Nature's Appeal Fading?

R. E. Bohn, J. E. Short, *How Much Information? 2009 Report on American Consumers*, Global Information Industry Center, University of California, San Diego, 2010.

"Cellphone Use Linked to Selfish Behavior," *ScienceDaily*, February 14, 2012 (see www.sciencedaily.com/releases/2012/02/120214122038.htm).

Convention on Biological Diversity (Cbd) & Airbus, *Bio-Index Report 2010* (see https://www.cbd.int/doc/groups/youth/greenwave/greenwave-airbus-bio-index-rep-2010-en.pdf).

Internet Access: Households and Individuals: 2015, Office for National Statistics, Newport. U.K., 2015 (see https://www.ons.gov.uk/peoplepopulation andcommunity/householdcharacteristics/home internet andsocialmediausage/bulletins/internetaccesshouseholds andindividuals/2015-08-06).

F. E. Kuo, "Parks and Other Green Environments: Essential Components of a Healthy Human Habitat; Executive Summary," National Recreation and Park Association, Ashburn, VA, 2010.

F. E. Kuo, W. C. Sullivan, "Environment and Crime in the Inner City: Does Vegetation Reduce Crime?" *Environment and Behavior* 33(3), 2001: 343–67.

Level of Internet Access: Households, Eurostat 2016 (see http://ec.europa.eu/eurostat/tgm/table.do?tab=table&init=1&plugin=1&language=en&pcode= tin00134).

Q. Li et al., "Relationships Between Percentage of Forest Coverage and Standardized Mortality Ratios (SMR) of Cancers in All Prefectures in Japan," *The Open Public Health Journal* 1, 2008: 1–7.

A. Perrin, *Social Media Usage: 2005–2015*, Pew Research Center, 2015 (see http://www.pewinternet.org/2015/10/08/social-networking-usage-2005-2015/).

J. Schipperijn et al., "Factors Influencing the Use of Green Space: Results from a Danish National Representative Survey," *Landscape and Urban Planning* 95, 2010: 130–37.

E. M. Selhub, A. C. Logan, *Your Brain on Nature: The Science of Nature's Influence on Your Health, Happiness and Vitality* (Hoboken, NJ: Wiley, 2014).

J. E. Short, *How Much Media? 2013 Report on American Consumers*, Institute for Communications Technology Management, Marshall School of Business, University of Southern California, San Diego, 2013.

U. K. Stigsdotter et al., "Health Promoting Outdoor Environments: Associations Between Green Space, and Health, Health-related Quality of Life and Stress Based on a Danish National Representative Survey," *Scandinavian Journal of Public Health* 38(4), 2010: 411–17.

3: Stress, Immune Defenses, and the Experience of Nature

American Psychological Association, *Stress in America: Our Health at Risk*, Washington, D.C., 2012 (see https://www.apa.org/news/press /releases/stress/2011/final-2011.pdf).

American Psychological Association, *Stress in America: Paying with Our Health*, Washington, D.C., 2015 (see https://www.apa.org/news /press/releases/stress/2014/stress-report.pdf).

American Psychological Association, *Stress in America: Coping with Change—Part 1*, Washington, D.C., 2017 (see https://www.apa.org /news/press/releases/stress/2016/coping-with-change.pdf).

F. Bottaccioli, *Il sistema immunitario: la bilancia della vita* (Milan: Tecniche nuove, 2008).

D. Dragoş, M. D. Tănăsescu, "The Effect of Stress on the Defense Systems," *Journal of Medicine and Life* 3(1), 2010: 10–18.

European Agency for Safety and Health at Work, *OSH in Figures: Stress at Work—Facts and Figures*, European Communities, Luxembourg, 2009.

P. Grahn, U. K. Stigsdotter, "Landscape Planning and Stress," *Urban Forestry Urban Greening* 2, 2003: 1–18.

M. Grandi, *Immunologia e fitoterapia* (Milan: Tecniche nuove, 2008).

A. Holbrook, *The Green We Need: An Investigation of the Benefits of Green Life and Green Spaces for Urban-Dwellers' Physical, Mental and Social Health* (Newcastle, Australia: University of Newcastle, 2009).

L. E. Keniger et al., "What Are the Benefits of Interacting with Nature?" *International Journal of Environmental Research and Public Health* 10(3), 2013: 913–35.

J. LeDoux, *The Emotional Brain: The Mysterious Underpinnings of Emotional Life* (New York: Simon & Schuster, 1996) (trad. it. *Il cervello emotivo. Alle origini delle emozioni* [Milan: Baldini & Castoldi, 1998]).

R. S. Ulrich, "View Through a Window May Influence Recovery from Surgery," *Science* 224, 1984: 420–21.

4: The Therapeutic Landscape

G. Bateson, *Mind and Nature: A Necessary Unity* (London: Wildwood, 1979).

Dentamaro et al., "Valutazione del potenziale rigenerativo di tipologie distinte di spazi verdi urbani e periurbani," *Forest@8*, 2011, 162–78 (see http://www.sisef.it/forest@/contents/?id=efor0673-008).

J. H. Falk, J. D. Balling, "Evolutionary Influence on Human Landscape Preference," *Environment and Behavior* 42 (4), 2010: 479–93.

W. M. Gesler, *Healing Places* (Oxford, U.K.: Rowman & Littlefield, 2003).

P. Grahn, U. K. Stigsdotter, "What Makes a Garden a Healing Garden?" *Journal of Therapeutic Horticulture* 13, 2002: 60–69.

T. Hartig et al., "A Measure of Restorative Quality in Environments," *Scandinavian Housing & Planning Research* 14, 1997: 175–94.

P. Inghilleri, N. Rainisio, "I luoghi del benessere. I parchi tra strategie cognitive ed empowerment territoriale," in G. Scaramellini, ed., *Paesaggi, territori, culture. Viaggio nei luoghi e nelle memorie del Parco del Ticino* (Milan: Cisalpino Editore, 2010), 219–50.

Y. Joye, A. E. Van Den Berg, "Is Love for Green in Our Genes?: A Critical Analysis of Evolutionary Assumptions in Restorative Environments Research," *Urban Forestry & Urban Greening* 10(4), 2011: 261–68.

Y. Joye, A. E. Van Den Berg, "Restorative Environments," in L. Steg et al. (ed.), *Environmental Psychology: An Introduction* (London: Wiley, 2012), 57–66.

S. Kaplan, "The Restorative Benefits of Nature: Towards an Integrative Framework," *Journal of Environmental Psychology* 15, 1995: 169–82.

S. Kaplan, R. Kaplan, "Health, Supportive Environments, and the Reasonable Person Model," *American Journal of Public Health* 93(9), 2003: 1484–89.

K. Laumann et al., "Rating Scale Measures of Restorative Components of Environments," *Journal of Environmental Psychology* 21(1), 2001: 31–44.

V. I. Lohr, "Benefits of Nature: What We Are Learning About Why People Respond to Nature," *Journal of Physiological Anthropology* 26(2), 2007: 83–85.

V. I. Lohr, C. H. Pearson-Mims, "Responses to Scenes with Spreading, Rounded and Conical Tree Forms," *Environment and Behavior* 38 (5), 2006: 667–88.

P. Pradhan, *The Role of Water as a Restorative Component in Small Urban Spaces* (Uppsala: Swedish University of Agricultural Sciences, 2012).

U. K. Stigsdotter et al., "Nature-Based Therapeutic Interventions," in K. Nilsson et al., eds., *Forests, Trees and Human Health* (New York: Springer, 2011), 309–42.

J. Summit, R. Sommer, "Further Studies of Preferred Tree Shapes," *Environment and Behavior* 31(4), 1999: 550–76.

A. Williams, "Therapeutic Landscapes in Holistic Medicine," *Social Science & Medicine* 46(9), 1998: 1193–1203.

Online

http://www.laragnaia.com/IT/intro/

5: Forest Bathing

H. H. Bartelink, "Allometric Relationships for Biomass and Leaf Area of Beech (*Fagus sylvatica L.*)," *Annales des Sciences Forestières* 54(1), 1997: 39–50.

N. Bertin et al., "Diurnal and Seasonal Course of Monoterpene Emissions from *Quercus ilex* (L.) Under Natural Conditions Application of Light and Temperature Algorithms," *Atmospheric Environment* 31 (suppl. 1), 1997: 135–44.

G. Bertini et al., "Densità di biomassa e necromassa legnosa in cedui invecchiati di leccio in Sardegna e di faggio in Toscana," *Forest@* 9, 2012: 108–29.

G. Calamini, E. Gregori, "Studio di una faggeta dell'appennino pistolese: relazioni allometriche per la stima della biomassa epigea," *L'Italia forestale e montana* 1, 2001: 1–23.

T. Dindorf et al., "Significant Light and Temperature Dependent Monoterpene Emissions from European Beech (*Fagus sylvatica L.*) and Their Potential Impact on the European Volatile Organic Compound Budget," *Journal of Geophysical Research* 111, 2006: 1–15.

C. Geron et al., "A Review and Synthesis of Monoterpene Speciation from Forests in the United States," *Atmospheric Environment* No. 34, 2000: 1761–81.

A. Guenther et al., "Natural Volatile Compound Emission Rate Estimates for U.S. Woodland Landscapes," *Atmospheric Environment* 28(6), 1994: 1197–1210.

M. Karl et al., "A New European Plant-Specific Emission Inventory of Biogenic Volatile Organic Compounds for Use in Atmospheric Transport Models," *Biogeosciences* 6, 2009: 1059–87.

T. Keenan et al., "Process Based Inventory of Isoprenoid Emissions from European Forests: Model Comparisons, Current Knowledge and Uncertainties," *Atmospheric Chemistry and Physics* 9(12), 2009: 4053–76.

J. Kesselmeier, M. Staudt, "Biogenic Volatile Organic Compounds (VOC): An Overview on Emission, Physiology and Ecology," *Journal of Atmospheric Chemistry* 33(1), 1999: 23–88.

J. Lee et al., "Nature Therapy and Preventive Medicine," in J. Maddock, ed., *Public Health. Social and Behavioral Health* (Maastricht: Institute for New Technologies, 2012) 325–50.

Q. Li, "Effect of Forest Bathing Trips on Human Immune Function," *Environmental Health and Preventive Medicine* 15, 2010: 9–17.

Q. Li et al., "Phytoncide (Wood Essential Oils) Induce Human Natural Killer Cell Activity," *Immunopharmacology and Immunotoxicology* 28, 2006: 319–33.

J. Llusià, J. Peñuelas, "Seasonal Patterns of Terpene Content and Emission from Seven Mediterranean Woody Species in Field Conditions," *American Journal of Botany* 87(1), 2000: 133–40.

S. N. Matsunaga et al., "Monoterpene and Sesquiterpene Emissions from Sugi (*Cryptomeria japonica*) Based on a Branch Enclosure Measurements," *Atmospheric Pollution Research* 2(1), 2011: 16–23.

S. Owen et al., "Screening of 18 Mediterranean Plant Species for Volatile Organic Compound Emissions," *Atmospheric Environment* 31 (suppl. 1), 1997: 101–17.

B. Park et al., "Physiological Effects of Forest Recreation in a Young Conifer Forest in Hinokage Town, Japan," *Silva Fennica* 43(2), 2009: 291–301.

B. Park et al., "The Physiological Effects of Shinrin-yoku (Taking In the Forest Atmosphere or Forest Bathing): Evidence from Field Experiments in 24 Forests Across Japan," *Environmental Health and Preventive Medicine* 15(1), 2010: 18–26.

B. Park et al., "Physiological Effects of Shinrin-yoku (Taking In the Atmosphere of the Forest) Using Salivary Cortisol and Cerebral Activity as Indicators," *Journal of Physiological Anthropology* 26(2), 2007: 123–28.

R. A. Street et al., "Effect of Habitat and Age on Variations in Volatile Organic Compound (VOC) Emissions from *Quercus ilex* and *Pinus pinea*," *Atmospheric Environment* 31 (suppl. 1), 1997: 89–100.

Y. Tsunetsugu et al., "Physiological Effects of Shinrin-yoku (Taking In the Atmosphere of the Forest) in an Old-Growth Broadleaf Forest in Yamagata Prefecture, Japan," *Journal of Physiological Anthropology* 26(2), 2007: 135–42.

Y. Tsunetsugu et al., "Trend in Research Related to 'Shinrin-yoku' (Taking In the Forest Atmosphere or Forest Bathing) in Japan," *Environmental Health and Preventive Medicine* 15(1), 2010: 27–37.

Q. Zheng, X. Yang, "Study and Practice of Forest-bathing Field in Japan," *Asian Journal of Agricultural Research* 5(2), 2013: 18–20, 25.

6: Negative Ions and Natural Environments

R. A. Baron, "Effects of Negative Ions on Cognitive Performance," *Journal of Applied Psychology* 72(1), 1987: 131–37.

M. Ehn et al., "Composition and Temporal Behavior of Ambient Ions in the Boreal Forest," *Atmospheric Chemistry and Physics* 10(17), 2010: 8513–30.

J.-L. Guilmot, ed., *Effets bénéfiques de l'ionisation négative de l'air. Revue de 70 publications scientifiques (1975–2010)*, Air Plus Environnement, s.l. 2011 (see http://www.ionisation.be/Effets_benefiques _de_l_ionisation_negative_de_l_air_Revue_de_70_publications _scientifiques_Mars_2011.pdf).

P. Kolarž et al., "Characterization of Ions at Alpine Waterfalls," *Atmospheric Chemistry and Physics* 12(8), 2012: 3687–97.

A. P. Krueger, E. J. Reed, "Biological Impact of Small Air Ions," *Science* 193(4259), 1976: 1209–13.

E. R. Jayaratne, "Trees Are Changing the Air You Breathe, but Not in the Way You Think," *The Conversation*, April 9, 2012 (see http://theconversation.com/trees-are-changing-the-air-you-breathe-but-not-in-the-way-you-think-6119).

E. R. Jayaratne et al., "Role of Vegetation in Enhancing Radon Concentration and Ion Production in the Atmosphere," *Environmental Science & Technology* 45(15), 2011: 6350–55.

"New Concerns About Ionizing Air Cleaners," *Consumer Reports* 5, 2005: 22–25.

Nikken Research Institute, *White Paper. Negative Ions: A Beneficial Atmospheric Phenomenon* (see http://www.nikkensleepcenter.com/information/NRI_negative-ion.pdf).

O. Pino, F. La Ragione, "There's Something in the Air: Empirical Evidence for the Effects of Negative Air Ions (NAI) on Psycho-physiological State and Performance," *Research in Psychology and Behavioral Sciences* 1(4), 2013: 48–53.

M. Scalia et al., *Ioni aerei e salute umana*, ed. F. Pulcini (Rome: Andromeda, 2013).

7: The Bioenergetic Landscape

G. Ananda, *Quando l'acqua sognava di volare. L'elettromagnetismo nel prisma dell'antenna Lecher* (Vicenza: AltroMondo Editore, 2016).

E. Bach, *I fiori che guariscono l'anima* (Milan: Tea Edizioni, 2003).

C. Backster, *Primary Perception: Biocommunication with Plants, Living Foods, and Human Cells* (Anza, CA: White Rose Millennium Press, 2003).

F. Baluška, S. Mancuso, "Vision in Plants via Plant-Specific Ocelli?" *Trends in Plant Science* 21(9), 2016: 727–30.

P. Bellavite, *Biodinamica. Basi fisiopatologiche e tracce di metodo per una medicina integrata* (Milan: Tecniche nuove, 1998).

J. C. Bose, *Response in the Living and Non-Living* (London and New York: Longmans, Green, 1902).

J. C. Bose, *The Nervous Mechanisms of Plants* (London and New York: Longmans, Greens, 1926).

J. Brosse, *Mythologie des arbres* (Paris: Payot, 1993) (trad. it. *Mitologia degli alberi. Dal giardino dell'Eden al legno della croce* [Milan: Rizzoli, 2000]).

S. H. Bunher, *The Lost Language of Plants: The Ecological Importance of Plant Medicine to Life on Earth* (White River Junction, VT: Chelsea Green Publishing, 2013).

H. S. Burr, *Blueprint for Immortality: The Electric Patterns of Life* (London: Neville Spearman, 1972).

F. Capra, *The Tao of Physics: An Exploration of the Parallels Between Modern Physics and Eastern Mysticism* (Boulder, CO: Shambhala, 1975).

D. Chamovitz, *What a Plant Knows* (New York: Farrar, Straus and Giroux, 2012).

M. Ceruti, E. Laszlo, eds., *Physis: abitare la terra* (Milan: Feltrinelli, 1988).

C. R. Darwin, *The Power of Movement in Plants* (New York: Da Capo Press, 1966).

P. Debertolis, D. Gullà, "Anthropological Analysis of Human Body Emissions Using New Photographic Technologies," *Proceedings in*

Scientific Conference: The 3rd International Virtual Conference on Advanced Scientific Results (SCIE-CONF-2015) 3(1), 2015: 162–68.

V. B. Dröscher, *Magie der Sinne im Tierreich. Neue Forschungen* (Monaco: List, 1966) (trad. it. *Magia dei sensi nel mondo animale* [Milan: Feltrinelli, 1968]).

M. Eliade, *Le sacré et le profane* (Paris: Gallimard, 1967) (trad. it. *Il sacro e il profano* [Turin: Boringhieri, 1967]).

G. J. Frazer, *The Golden Bough* (London: Macmillan, 1890) (trad. it. *Il ramo d'oro* [Turin: Einaudi, 1950]).

H. Frohlich, *Biological Coherence and Response to External Stimuli* (Heidelberg: Springer, 1988).

M. Gagliano, "Green Symphonies: A Call for Studies on Acoustic Communication in Plants," *Behavioral Ecology* 24(4), 2013: 789–96.

M. Gagliano, "The Mind of Plants: Thinking the Unthinkable," *Communicative and Integrative Biology* 10(2), 1288333, 17 Feb. 2017, doi.10.1080/19420889.2017.1288333.

M. Gagliano et al., "Learning by Association in Plants," *Scientific Report* 6, 38427, 2016.

M. Gagliano et al., "Plants Learn and Remember: Let's Get Used to It," *Oecologia* 186, 2018, 29–31.

R. Gerber, *Vibrational Medicine: New Choices for Healing Ourselves* (Santa Fe: Bear & Company, 1988).

E. M. Goodman et al., "Effects of Electromagnetic Fields on Molecules and Cells," *International Review of Cytology* 158, 1995: 279–339.

H. Hesse, *Stunden im Garte. Eine Idylle* (Vienna: Bermann-Fischer, 1936) (trad. it. *In giardino* [Parma: Guanda, 1994]).

H. l'Arpenteur, *L'établissement des limites*, ed. M. Clavel-Lévêque et al. (Naples: Jovene, 1996) (*Corpus agrimensorum romanorum*, 4).

C. G. Jung, *Die Archetypen und das kollektive Unbewusste* (Zurich: Rascher, 1976) (trad. it. *Gli archetipi e l'inconscio collettivo* [Turin: Boringhieri, 1980]).

C. G. Jung, *Der philosophische Baum* (Basel, 1945) (trad. it. *L'albero filosofico* [Turin: Boringhieri, 1983]).

K. G. Korotkov, *Human Energy Field: Study with GDV Bioelectrography* (Lancaster, PA: Backbone, 2002).

K. G. Korotkov, *Kirlian Effect* (St. Petersburg: Olga Publishing House, 1995).

W. A. Kunnen et al., *Il corpo energetico dell'uomo e la biosfera secondo Walter Kunnen. L'approccio energetico in biologia e medicina, magnetoterapia ed antenna Lecher* (Rome: Andromeda, 2012).

B. H. Lipton, *The Biology of Belief: Unleashing the Power of Consciousness, Matter & Miracles* (Carlsbad, CA: Hay House, 2005) (trad. it. *La biologia delle credenze. Come il pensiero influenza il DNA e ogni cellula* [Cesena: Macro edizioni, 2012]).

B. H. Lipton, *La mente è più forte dei geni. La nuova scienza che ci restituisce i nostri poteri* (Cesena: Macro edizioni, 2007).

J. Lovelock, *The Ages of Gaia: A Biography of Our Living Earth* (Oxford, U.K.: Oxford University Press, 1989) (trad. it. *Le nuove età di Gaia* [Turin: Bollati Boringhieri, 1991]).

S. Mancuso, *Botanica: Viaggio nell'universo vegetale*, Aboca edizionié, Sansepolcro, 2017.

S. Mancuso, *Plant revolution: Le piante hanno già scritto il nostro futuro* (Florence: Giunti, 2017).

S. Mancuso, F. Baluška, "Plant Ocelli for Visually Guided Plant Behavior," *Trends in Plants Science* 22, 2017: 5–6.

S. Mancuso, A. Viola, *Verde brillante: Sensibilità e intelligenza del mondo vegetale* (Florence: Giunti, 2013).

P. Manzelli et al., *I segreti dell'acqua. L'opera scientifica di Giorgio Piccardi* (Rome: Di Renzo Editore, 1994).

J. Monro et al., "Electrical Sensitivities in Allergic Patients," *Clinical Ecology* 4(3), 1987: 93–102.

M. Nieri, "Bioenergetic Landscapes: An Innovative Technique to Create Effective 'Healing Gardens' Utilizing the Beneficial Electromagnetic Properties of Plants," *ISHS Acta Horticulturae* 881, 2010: 859–62.

M. Nieri, *Bioenergetic Landscape: La progettazione del giardino terapeutico bioenergetico* (Naples: Sistemi Editoriali, 2009).

M. Nieri, A. Zechini D'Aulerio, *Indagine con misurazioni e.m. sullo stato sanitario di piante arboree in un Parco a Bologna*, 2004 (unpublished report).

G. L. Playfair, S. Hill, *The Cycles of Heaven* (New York: Avon, 1979) (trad. it. *Gli influssi del cosmo sulla vita terrestre* [Turin: MEB, 1981]).

M. Pollan, *The Botany of Desire* (New York: Random House, 2001).

M. Pollan, "The Intelligent Plant," *The New Yorker,* Dec. 23, 2013.

F. A. Popp, *Biologie des Lichts. Grundlagen der ultraschwachen Zellstrahlun* (Berlino-Amburgo: Parey, 1984).

F. A. Popp, *Neue Horizonte in der Medizin* (Heidelberg: Haug, 1983) (trad. it *Nuovi orizzonti in medicina: La teoria dei biofotoni* [Palermo: Ipsa, 1985]).

V. Rajda, *Electrodiagnostics of the Health of Oak Trees* (Brno: CSAV, 1992).

R. E. Rockwell et al., *Hug a Tree and Other Things to Do Outdoors with Young Children* (Mt. Rainer, MD: Gryphon House, 1983).

R. Sheldrake, *A New Science of Life: The Hypothesis of Formative Causation* (London: Blond and Briggs, 1981).

C. W. Smith, S. Best, *Electromagnetic Man: Health and Hazard in the Electrical Environment* (London: Dent, 1990).

U. K. Stigsdotter, P. Grahn, "A Garden at Your Workplace May Reduce Stress," *Design & Health III* (Stockholm, 2004): 147–57.

A. Szent-Györgyi, *Bioelectronics: A Study in Cellular Regulations, Defense, and Cancer* (New York: Academic Press, 1968).

Teofrasto di Ereso, *La storia delle piante*, ed. F. Ferri Mancini (Rome: Loescher, 1900).

N. Tesla, *My Inventions* (La Jolla, CA: Stefan University Press, 2008) (trad. it. *Le mie invenzioni. Autobiografia di un genio* [Prato: Piano B, 2012]).

P. Tompkins, C. Bird, *The Secret Life of Plants* (London: Penguin, 1972) (trad. it. *La vita segreta delle piante* [Milan: Il Saggiatore, 2002]).

C. Ventura, L. Tavazzi, "Biophysical Signalling from and to the (Stem) Cells: A Novel Path to Regenerative Medicine," *European Journal of Heart Failure* 18, 2016: 1405–07.

C. Ventura, "Fashioning Cellular Rhythms with Magnetic Energy and Sound Vibration: A New Perspective for Regenerative Medicine," *CellR4* 2(2), 2014: 839.

C. Weaver, R. D. Astumian, "The Response of Living Cells to Very Weak Electric Fields: The Thermal Noise Limit," *Science* 247, 1990: 459–62.

E. Zürcher et al., "Fasi lunari e proprietà del legno. Una sperimentazione sull'effetto della data di abbattimento," *Sherwood* 163, 2010: 13–17.

Online

Archibo Biologica (Belgio): www.archibo-biologica.be.

HeartMath Institute: www.heartmath.org.

LINV International Laboratory of Plant Neurobiology: www.linv .org.

Primary Perception (intervista a Cleve Backster su percezione primaria e biocomunicazione): https://www.youtube.com/watch?v= V7V6D33HGt8.

VID Art-Science, fondata da Carlo Ventura: vidartscience.org.

8: Air-Purifying Indoor Plants

J. C. Allen et al., "Associations of Cognitive Function Scores with Carbon Dioxide, Ventilation, and Volatile Organic Compound Exposures in Office Workers: A Controlled Exposure Study of Green and Conventional Office Environments," *Environmental Health Perspectives* 124(6), 2016: 805–12.

Ambient Air Pollution: A Global Assessment of Exposure and Burden of Disease (Geneva: World Health Organization, 2016).

W. R. Bastos et al., "Mercury Persistence in Indoor Environments in the Amazon Region, Brazil," *Environmental Research* 96 (2004): 235–38.

L. Brighigna et al., "The Use of Tropical Bromeliads (*Tillandsia* spp.) for Monitoring Atmospheric Pollution in the Town of Florence, Italy," *Revista de Biologia Tropical* 50(2), 2002: 577–84.

T. Bringslimark et al., "Psychological Benefits of Indoor Plants in Workplaces: Putting Experimental Results into Context," *HortScience* 42(3), 2007: 581–87.

C. Y. Chang, P. K. Chen, "Human Response to Window Views and Indoor Plants in the Workplace," *HortScience* 40(5), 2005: 1354–59.

P. Costa, R. W. James, "Constructive Use of Vegetation in Office Buildings," presented at the Plants for People Symposium, The Hague, Netherlands, November 23, 1995.

A. Dravigne et al., "The Effect of Live Plants and Window Views of Green Spaces on Employee Perceptions of Job Satisfaction," *Hort-Science* 43(1), 2008: 183–87.

M. Eliade, *Traité d'histoire des religions* (Paris: Payot, 1949) (trad. it. *Trattato di storia delle religioni* [Turin: Boringhieri, 1972]).

H. Fischer, *Stoff-Wechsel: Auf dem Weg zu einer solaren Chemie für das 2. Jahrhundert* (Munich: Kunstmann, 2012).

T. Fjeld, "The Effect of Interior Planting on Health and Discomfort Among Workers and School Children," *HortTechnology* 10(1), 2000: 46–52.

T. Fjeld, C. Bonnevie, "The Effect of Plants and Artificial Daylight on the Well-being and Health of Office Workers, School Children and Health Care Personnel," in *Seminar Report: Reducing Health Complaints at Work*, Plants for People, International Horticultural Exhibition Floriade, Amsterdam 2002.

M. Giese et al., "Detoxification of Formaldehyde by the Spider Plant (*Chlorophytum comosum L.*) and by Soybean (*Glycine max L.*) Cell-Suspension Cultures," *Plant Physiology* 104(4), 1994: 1301–1309.

J. R. Girman et al., "Critical Review: How Well Do Houseplants Perform as Indoor Air Cleaners?" *Proceedings of Healthy Buildings* 23, 2009: 667–72.

T. Higa, *An Earth-Saving Revolution: A Means to Resolve Our World's Problems Through Effective Microorganisms* (Tokyo: Sunmark, 1996) (trad. it. *Microrganismi effettivi, benessere e rigenerazione nel rispetto della natura* [Milan: Tecniche nuove, 2006]).

H. Ikei et al., "The Physiological and Psychological Relaxing Effects of Viewing Rose Flowers in Office Workers," *Journal of Physiological Anthropology (JSPA)* 33(1), 2014: 1–5.

S. R. Kellert et al., *Biophilic Design: The Theory, Science and Practice of Bringing Buildings to Life* (New York: Wiley, 2008).

K. J. Kim et al., "Efficiency of Volatile Formaldehyde Removal by Indoor Plants. Contribution of Aerial Plant Parts Versus the Root Zone," *Journal of the American Society for Horticultural Science* 133(4), 2008: 521–26.

V. I. Lohr et al., "Interior Plants May Improve Worker Productivity and Reduce Stress in a Windowless Environment," *Journal of Environmental Horticulture* 14 (2), 1996: 97–100.

V. I. Lohr, C. H. Pearson-Mims, "Particulate Matter Accumulation on Horizontal Surfaces in Interiors: Influence of Foliage Plants," *Atmospheric Environment* 30(14), 1996: 2565–68.

R. Nakamura, E. Fujii, "Studies of the Characteristics of the Electroencephalogram When Observing Potted Plants: *Pelargonium Hortorum* 'Sprinter Red' and *Begonia evansiana*," *Technical Bulletin of the Faculty of Horticulture of Chiba University* 43, 1990: 177–83.

A. Nel et al., "Toxic Potential of Materials at the Nanolevel," *Science* 311, 2006: 622–27.

M. Nieuwenhuis et al., "The Relative Benefits of Green Versus Lean Office Space: Three Field Experiments," *Journal of Experimental Psychology: Applied* 20(3), 2014: 199–214.

V. Niri, "Selecting the Right Houseplant Could Improve Indoor Air (animation)," *American Chemical Society*, New Releases, 2016 (see https://www.youtube.com/watch?v=HdOibycDIA4&feature=youtu.be).

D. J. Novak et al., "Tree and Forest Effects on Air Quality and Human Health in the United States," *Environmental Pollution* 193, 2014: 119–29.

"Public Creativity Put to the Test in Chelsea Flower Show Psychology Experiment," University of Exeter, May 16, 2013 (see http://www.exeter.ac.uk/news/research/title_291041_en.html).

Regolamento UE n. 605/2014 della Commissione del 5 giugno 2014 (see http://eur-lex.europa.eu/legal-content/IT/ALL/?uri=CELEX: 32014R0605).

D. Sarigiannis et al., "Exposure to Major Volatile Organic Compounds and Carbonyls in European Indoor Environments and Associated Health Risk," *Environment International* 37(4), 2011: 743–65.

U. Satish et al., "Is CO_2 an Indoor Pollutant? Direct Effects of Low-to-Moderate CO_2 Concentrations on Human Decision-Making Performance," *Environmental Health Perspectives* 120(12), 2012: 1671–77.

C. A. Shoemaker et al., "Relationships Between Plants, Behaviour, and Attitudes in an Office Environment," *HortTechnology* 2(2), 1992: 205–6.

A. Smith et al., "Healthy, Productive Workplaces: Towards a Case for Interior Plantscaping," *Facilities* 29(5/6), 2011: 209–23.

I. Stewart, "Eden Project Plant-Air Test Hailed a Success," BBC, Sept. 19, 2011 (see http://www. bbc.com/news/uk-england-14970685).

R. S. Ulrich, "Health Benefits of Gardens in Hospitals," in *Seminar Report: Reducing Health Complaints at Work,* presented at the Plants for People Conference, Floriade International Horticultural Exhibition, Haarlemmermeerse Woods, 2002.

X. Wei et al., "Phylloremediation of Air Pollutants: Exploiting the Potential of Plant Leaves and Leaf-Associated Microbes," *Frontiers in Plant Science* 8, 2017: 1318.

M. B. Wilkins, *Plantwatching: How Plants Live, Feel and Work* (London: Macmillan, 1988) (trad. it. *I segreti delle piante. Come vivono, come si riproducono, come si adattano all'ambiente* [Novara: Istituto Geografico De Agostini, 1989]).

B. C. Wolverton, *How to Grow Fresh Air: 50 Houseplants That Purify Your Home or Office* (London: Penguin, 1997) (trad. it. *Amiche piante. 50 piante per purificare l'aria in casa e in ufficio* [Milan: Geo, 1998]).

B. C. Wolverton, J. D. Wolverton, "Plants and Soil Microorganisms: Removal of Formaldehyde, Xylene, and Ammonia from the Indoor Environment," *Journal of the Mississippi Academy of Sciences* 38(2), 1993: 11–15.

B. C. Wolverton et al., *Interior Landscape Plants for Indoor Air Pollution Abatement: Final Report* (Washington, D.C.: National Aeronautics and Space Administration, 1989).

R. A. Wood et al., "Potted-Plant/Growth Media Interactions and Capacities for Removal of Volatiles from Indoor Air," *Journal of Horticultural Science and Biotechnology* 77(1), 2002: 120–29.

R. A. Wood et al., "The Potted-Plant Microcosm Substantially Reduces Indoor Air VOC Pollution: I. Office Field-Study," *Water, Air, and Soil Pollution* 175(1), 2006: 163–80.

D. S. Yang et al., "Screening Indoor Plants for Volatile Organic Pollutant Removal Efficiency," *HortScience* 44(5), 2009: 1377–81.

D. S. Yang et al., "Volatile Organic Compounds Emanating from Indoor Ornamental Plants," *HortScience* 44(2), 2009: 396–400.

Online
Green Plants for Green Buildings: www.greenplantsforgreen buildings.org.

Human Space Global Report: humanspaces.com/global-report /the-global-impact-of-biophilic-design-in-the-workplace.

Innovative Plants Technology: www.plantscleanair.com.

Kamal Meattle: www.pbcnet.com/about/indoor-air-quality and www.youtube.com/watch?time_continue=1318&v=wUBrBLHYHaI (interview on YouTube).

NASA Stennis Space Center: https://www.nasa.gov/centers/stennis/home/index.html.

NIGZ-Werk (Nationaal Instituut voor Gezondheidsbevordering en Ziektepreventie): www.healthygreenatwork.org (campaign to bring plants into the workplace sponsored by the European Union, 2004).

INDEX

trees, physical contact with,
146, 148; study of physical
reactions within human
body during, 115, 117; "tree
hugging" and, 116–17,
131–33, 142, 148
trichloroethylene, 160, 170, 173
trust, in natural spaces, 62
TRV (Variable Resonance
Camera), 146

Ulrich, Roger, 15, 41–42
urban environments, 2, 3,
7–8, 10, 11–12, 13, 15,
72, 92, 93, 100, 152;
accessibility of green
spaces in, 66–67; benefits
of green spaces in, 24–26;
bioenergetic gardens in,
141; environmental neglect
and, 16; ion content in,
103, 105; kids in, averse
to natural settings, 16–17;
regenerative effectiveness
of natural environments
vs., 56, 85

vacation, tech habits and,
27–28, 30
VEFs (vegetable energy fields),
146
ventilation of interior spaces,
109, 156–57, 177

Ventura, Carlo, 120
vision: color green and, 11; eye's
antenna function and, 122;
threatening stimuli and,
11–12
visitor's mental power, 64–65
visual disturbances, 52
visual use of green space, 68,
69, 71
volatile organic compounds
(VOCs), 91–92, 154–55;
reduced by houseplants,
160–64, 168–69, 170–73

water: moving, ion showers
and, 110–13; purified by
plant roots, 160–61; in
therapeutic landscape, 71,
73
Wilson, Edward O., 13, 14
wireless communications, 147
Wolverton, Bill, 160–61, 168,
172
Wood, Ronald, 163
workplaces. *See* offices and
other workplaces
World Health Organization, 24,
152, 153

Zegna Oasis, Biella, Italy, 98,
144

ABOUT THE AUTHORS

MARCO MENCAGLI has a degree in agronomy and has been working in the field for over twenty-five years. He specializes in the design and maintenance of public parks and private gardens, as well as of paths and facilities for the enjoyment of sanctuaries and protected areas. For twelve years he collaborated with Ente Parco Regionale della Maremma (board of the Regional Park of Maremma) as agronomy consultant. For some time now he has been focusing on the more therapeutic aspects of plants and natural environments. He is also a landscaping consultant for many prestigious touristic facilities in Tuscany and Lazio.

MARCO NIERI is a bioresearcher and a specialist in eco-design and environmental protection. He is the creator of bioenergetic landscaping, an innovative technique to study the effects of plant bioelectromagnetism on the human body, and the designer of therapeutic landscapes both in Italy and abroad. He organizes guided visits in natural parks and forests, for a direct experience of the biological interactions with plants and of the healing effect of trees on our organism. He is the author of *Bioenergetic Landscape*.

JAMIE RICHARDS is a translator based in Milan, Italy. She holds an MFA in literary translation from the University of Iowa and a PhD in comparative literature from the University of Oregon, and her translations include works by Igiaba Scego, Matteo Bussola, Ermanno Cavazzoni, Giovanni Orelli, and Zerocalcare.